MCQs in Epidemiology and Community Medicine

MCQs in Epidemiology and Community Medicine

Hugh Tunstall-Pedoe

MA MD FRCP FRCPE FFCM

Professor of Cardiovascular Epidemiology and Senior Lecturer in Medicine, Ninewells Hospital and Medical School, University of Dundee; Honorary Specialist in Community Medicine and Honorary Cardiologist, Tayside Health Board

WCS Smith

MD MPH MFCM

Senior Epidemiologist, Cardiovascular Epidemiology Unit, and Honorary Senior Lecturer in Community Medicine, Ninewells Hospital and Medical School, University of Dundee; Honorary Specialist in Community Medicine, Tayside Health Board

Churchill Livingstone ⣿

EDINBURGH LONDON MELBOURNE AND NEW YORK 1987

CHURCHILL LIVINGSTONE
Medical Division of Longman Group UK Limited

Distributed in the United States of America by Churchill
Livingstone Inc., 1560 Broadway, New York, N.Y. 10036,
and by associated companies, branches and
representatives throughout the world.

First published 1987

ISBN   0-443-03194-0

British Library Cataloguing in Publication Data
Pedoe, Hugh Tunstall
   MCQs in epidemiology and community
   medicine.
   1. Epidemiology — Problems, exercises, etc
   I. Title II. Smith, W.C.S.
   614.4'076   RA651

Library of Congress Cataloging in Publication Data Pedoe,
Hugh Tunstall.
MCQs in epidemiology and community medicine.
1. Epidemiology — Examinations, questions, etc. 2. Public
health — Examinations, questions, etc. 3. Epidemiology
— Great Britain — Examinations, questions, etc. 4. Public
health — Great Britain — Examinations, questions, etc. I.
Smith, W. C. S. (William Cairns Stewart) II. Title. [DNLM:
1. Community Medicine — examination questions. 2.
Epidemiology — examination questions. W 18 P371m]
RA652.7.P43   1987   614.4'076   87–8021

Produced by Longman Singapore Publishers (Pte) Ltd.
Printed in Singapore.

Preface

These questions follow a common pattern for British multiple choice questions in that each stem question is followed by five branches, each of which constitutes, with the stem, a complete statement in itself. Each branch can be true or false and the branches attached to each stem are largely independent of each other. There can be five true branches, five false ones or anything in between for each question, but in the long run the numbers of true and false statements are similar, and there is no regular pattern otherwise.

There are 110 questions altogether, constituting 550 statements. These have been organized into five papers, each of 22 questions. The questions for each paper are followed by answers with detailed explanations, so that the student can test his progress with the subject as learning or revision proceeds, and use the detailed answers to improve his or her knowledge of the subject. The level of knowledge tested by these questions is quite comprehensive, so we expect them to be used not only by undergraduates, but also by those working for the Faculty of Community Medicine examinations, by MPH students and by clinicians taking the increasingly popular courses in Epidemiology for Clinicians. Overall scoring is more important than difficulties with specific questions, but the authors would be pleased to hear about any ambiguities or disagreements, whether from students or from fellow teachers.

Each paper of 22 questions contains six on principles of epidemiology which are testing knowledge of concepts, six on specific epidemiology of common or topical chronic diseases, five on health services and five on infectious diseases and prevention. The answers are applicable to the United Kingdom in the 1980s. Readers from other countries may well find that most of the questions are very relevant to them but the answers may differ in detail, on occasion, with regard to the relative importance of different conditions. The organization of health services does differ from country to country so non-British readers should use these questions as a challenge to find out what they know about their own country. As the years go by some of the specifically British answers may be outdated by changing disease trends or further health service reorganization, but the book may have been revised by then.

We make no excuse for a number of questions on specific disease epidemiology. This is in danger of falling between two stools, so that it does not appear either in the syllabus for clinical teaching or in that for community medicine. The epidemiology of chronic diseases is of great interest and importance. Infectious disease epidemiology is now experiencing a rebirth and this is reflected in the questions on it.

We would like to thank Professor Charles Florey of the Department of Community Medicine of Dundee University and Dr Iain Crombie, Senior Statistician of the Cardiovascular Epidemiology Unit, for their helpful comments; responsibility for any remaining errors or ambiguities remains with the authors.

Dundee   Hugh Tunstall-Pedoe
1986   WCS Smith

Contents

Paper One — Questions

1.1 **Mortality rates in two different populations can be validly compared using**
- **A** mean age at death
- **B** proportion of the population over 65
- **C** numbers of deaths in each age group
- **D** life expectancy at birth
- **E** standardized mortality ratios (SMRs)

1.2 **In any given screening test**
- **A** the specificity is the percentage of truly negative subjects correctly classified by the test
- **B** the higher the specificity the lower the sensitivity
- **C** a low specificity means a spuriously high measured prevalence rate
- **D** high repeatability does not guarantee high validity
- **E** high sensitivity means few false negatives

1.3 **The incidence rate of a disease can be estimated directly from**
- **A** the proportion of hospital discharges with that diagnosis
- **B** the mortality rate if case fatality is very high
- **C** a cross-sectional population survey
- **D** first admission rates for diseases which always lead to hospital admission
- **E** logging of new cases in general practices with age-sex registers

1.4   Eight babies with spina bifida were reportedly born to women with hair dyed blonde and two to women using other hair dyes. It can be concluded that

A   there is a causal relationship between blonde hair dye and spina bifida

B   there is an association between the use of blonde hair dye and spina bifida

C   women who dye their hair blonde are more likely to become pregnant

D   a randomized controlled trial is justified

E   further information might be obtained from a case-control study

1.5   Crude birth rates in a country will fall if

A   life expectancy increases

B   divorce is legalized

C   the legal age of marriage is raised

D   house mortgage rates fall

E   the average spacing between babies increases

1.6   In a double-blind randomized clinical trial

A   nobody knows who is getting the active treatment

B   analysis should be based only on those who actually received the treatments concerned

C   patients should be blinded to the fact that they are in a trial

D   there must always be a placebo treatment

E   established drugs need not be monitored for side effects

1.7   Most coronary deaths occur

A   from acute myocardial infarction potentially demonstrable at necropsy

B   in subjects on long-term treatment for ischaemic heart disease

C   in hospital

D   in subjects below the age of 60

E   in persons with moderate or severe hypertension or hypercholesterolaemia

1.8   The risk of coronary heart disease from smoking cigarettes

A   shows the greatest relative risk in the younger age groups

B   appears to be reversible in those who stop smoking

C   accounts for as many smoking related deaths as does lung cancer

D   has a greater relative risk than does smoking for lung cancer

E   operates in populations with very low serum cholesterol levels

1.9 Lung cancer rates are increased in

A oil refinery workers
B the east end of major cities
C asbestos workers
D those exposed to arsenicals
E salt miners

1.10 Mortality rates from cirrhosis of the liver

A are lower in doctors than in other professional groups
B have increased in Britain over the last 30 years
C are particularly high in occupational groups which make extensive use of hospitality
D correlate with population mean alcohol consumption
E show no correlation with the real price of alcohol over time

1.11 Childhood rickets

A reached a peak of incidence in Britain with food rationing in World War II
B now occurs in Britain particularly in Asian immigrant families
C presents most commonly in early autumn
D can occur for dietary reasons other than vitamin D content
E occurred mostly in industrial towns at high latitudes

1.12 Diabetes mellitus

A is easily defined for clinical and epidemiological purposes
B prevalence increases with age
C confers a reduced life expectancy despite treatment
D usually causes death through its specific complications
E occurs only in industrialized, sedentary, Western populations

1.13 Morbidity data in the UK is routinely collected for statistical analysis

A from patients on admission to hospital
B from patients at out-patients attendance
C at general practitioner consultations
D on diagnosis of new cancers
E in the General Household Survey

1.14 The World Health Organization (WHO)

A has its headquarters in New York
B is funded on a similar basis to the United Nations
C was largely responsible for co-ordinating the efforts to eradicate smallpox
D does not produce any publications by itself
E is concerned only with communicable diseases and environmental health

1.15 Health authorities in the UK are responsible for
  A   Social Work Departments
  B   primary health care
  C   Environmental Health Department
  D   social security
  E   community dentistry

1.16 Expenditure in the National Health Service (NHS)
  A   is mostly on staff salaries
  B   on salaries is mostly to pay doctors
  C   is mostly on hospital services
  D   is greater on acute services than on long-term care
  E   on capital projects has no effect on recurring expenditure

1.17 Health information
  A   services are provided in each health authority
  B   from claims for sickness benefit are of limited value
  C   services collect details of hospital bed usage
  D   services are essential for health service planning
  E   on cancer incidence is collected by cancer registries

1.18 Disease notification
  A   is a reliable source of information about infectious diseases
  B   is the same in most countries
  C   of cholera is required in all countries
  D   can be encouraged by financial incentives
  E   of infectious disease requires laboratory evidence

1.19 Measles
  A   deaths are usually caused by secondary pneumonia
  B   infection has a high case fatality rate in developing countries
  C   incidence is not dramatically changed by use of the vaccine
  D   vaccine is usually given at the age of five years
  E   vaccine is usually given as a single dose

1.20 Malaria
  A   prophylaxis is always effective
  B   prophylaxis should not be given in pregnancy
  C   resistance to chloroquine is common in SE Asia
  D   prophylaxis should be continued for one month after return
      from a malarial country
  E   misdiagnosed in a febrile patient from a malarial area is
      usually regarded as medical negligence

1.21 Health education is important

    A since health behaviour is closely related to level of knowledge

    B and makes up a large part of the secondary school curriculum

    C but is not very effective when given by a doctor

    D and health authorities usually have their own health education centres

    E but the benefits usually take a long time to become apparent

1.22 Adequate housing in the UK

    A is defined as a house meeting 'tolerable standards'

    B need not have a supply of hot water

    C should not have more than two persons per room

    D can have an outside toilet

    E is maintained by regular inspections by the health authority

Paper One — Answers

1.1 A **False**   This will be affected by the proportions of people at different ages, as well as the risks of death at different ages. A population which has been rapidly expanding by reproduction will have a small proportion of elderly people, and therefore a low mean age at death.

      B **False**   The same argument applies as above. In populations with identical birth rates over many years, and no migration in or out, mean age at death and the proportion of the population over 65 would reflect only differences in mortality. Birth rate and migration are major complicating factors.

      C **False**   Numbers of deaths in each age group will vary with the number at risk, the time period and the risk of death. There must be a standard denominator and time period to give a death rate.

      D **True**   Life expectancy at birth is calculated using the risk of death at different ages and is therefore a reasonable summary measure of differences in mortality between populations, although it will not show at which ages the differences are occurring.

      E **True**   Standardization implies that differences in age structure of the populations have been allowed for, even though the effects are not completely removed by the usual methods. SMRs are based on an expected value of 100 so that they are a relative, and not an absolute, measure of risk.

1.2 A True   That is how the specificity of a test is defined. 100% specificity means no false positives but 98% specificity means that 2% of all normal subjects screened will be falsely classified as cases.

B True   This is an inevitable result of moving the cut-off point in a test. Raising the threshold to reduce the number of false positives (increasing the specificity) will result in more true positives being classified falsely as negative, with a consequent reduction in sensitivity.

C True   The measured prevalence rate will be the proportion of positives among those screened. Low specificity means a high proportion of false positives so the apparent prevalence will be falsely high.

D True   While a test must be repeatable if it is valid, the converse is not necessarily true as it could be consistently measuring something else. (e.g. it might be claimed that weight in kilograms is conveniently estimated by halving the height in centimetres. The latter method would be highly repeatable in the answer it gave, but not valid).

E True   Sensitivity is the ability of the test to characterize true positives as positive, implying therefore few false negatives.

1.3 A **False** There are three major sources of error. The first is that it is only certain diseases that inevitably lead to hospital admission, the second that patients may be admitted several times for the same condition, and the third that the denominator for incidence is the population at risk and not the total of hospital admissions. This index could be called proportional discharge rate or ratio, or something similar, leaving incidence rate its specific meaning.

B **True** Mortality and incidence rates are conceptually similar (event rate per 100 000, or other, per year). While rabies is about the only disease with 100% fatality rate, it has been so close in certain cancers (e.g. stomach, bronchus) that mortality and incidence rates are interchangeable.

C **False** A cross-sectional study is carried out at one time. It can therefore be used to measure a prevalence rate, but not an incidence rate, which is the rate of occurrence of new cases over time. (Incidence rates may be estimated indirectly using changes by age in prevalence, for example, of previous history of, or antibodies to, infectious diseases of childhood).

D **True** Provided that the rates are based on population denominators and not hospital discharges (see A).

E **True** General practices with age-sex registers know the population at risk and are able to calculate incidence rates for those diseases which present to medical attention. Unfortunately, the size of a single practice list is too small to estimate incidence for any but really common complaints, so that collaborative studies are needed.

1.4 A False   The evidence given is inadequate. It would be necessary to know what numbers of women and of pregnancies were involved and what attempts had been made to exclude confounding factors before this could be postulated. Ideally similar results should be obtained from different sorts of studies carried out by different observers in different populations.

B False   On the evidence given it is not possible to state whether the number of abnormal pregnancies was greater or less than expected. Blonde dyes might be used much more commonly and in a younger age group than other dyes.

C False   On the evidence given it is not possible to state whether the number of pregnancies was greater or less than expected.

D False   It would be quite wrong to go to a trial in the absence of further information from case-control studies and cohort studies. In any case it is not ethical to carry out a randomized controlled trial of an agent that is considered potentially toxic, although it might be possible to do a trial of randomized withdrawal of the agent.

E True   A case-control study would be the quickest and simplest method of testing for an association and also looking for confounding factors. Mothers of spina bifida cases could be compared with mothers of normal pregnancies for use of hair dye, after matching for age, social class, parity and locality.

1.5 A True   As more people survive beyond the normal childbearing and child rearing ages they contribute to the denominator of the crude birth rate (births per 1000 all ages per year) and not to the numerator.

B False   Divorce and remarriage often leads to the starting of another brood of children.

C True   This is a method of population control. Compulsory male conscription with no home leave will have a similar effect.

D False   Mortgage rates have an inverse effect on the birth rate.

E True   As the spacing increases, the average size of the completed family falls.

1.6 A **False** Whilst it is true that neither the patient nor those making the end-point evaluations should know which treatment group the patient is in, analysis of results depends on somebody knowing, and the interim analysis of unwanted effects of the different therapies can only be done by someone who is not 'blinded'.

B **False** Patients are randomized on the intention to treat so that it is only the groups intended for the different treatments who are truly comparable. Once patients start to drop out the comparability is lost. Main analyses should therefore be done by the intention to treat, although secondary analyses can also be done on those who were actually receiving the different treatments.

C **False** Patients should be blinded as to which treatment they are receiving, but they should have given informed consent to their participation in the trial.

D **False** It is possible to compare two active treatments. Where there is an established effective treatment, any new treatment should be compared with that and not with an inactive one.

E **False** Established drugs may never have been subjected to a double blind assessment of their unwanted effects. When this was done for thiazide diuretic treatment of mild hypertension it was found that the side effects (such as impotence) were much more common than had previously been thought.

1.7 A **False** The majority of coronary deaths occur within a few minutes of the onset of symptoms and in these cases evidence of infarction is usually absent.

B **False** About half of the victims have some previous history of cardiovascular disease but most victims are not currently under treatment.

C **False** The majority of deaths occur out of hospital, although death certificates of victims brought in to hospital, already dead, may have the hospital named on them as the place of death.

D **False** Although coronary disease is a very major cause of premature death, some two thirds of male deaths occur above age 65 and the proportion in women is even higher.

E **False** A minority of coronary victims have markedly elevated levels of individual risk factors, whereas a large proportion have moderately elevated levels of more than one which are passed as 'normal' even though they are associated with increased multifactorial risk.

1.8 A **True**   The risk of a heavy smoker having a coronary compared with a non-smoker is at its greatest in the younger age groups where the effect is so strong that it is unusual to see non-smokers under 45 admitted to coronary care units.

   B **True**   Observational studies suggest that coronary risk in smokers becomes similar to that in non-smokers after 5 to 10 years, if they stop smoking completely.

   C **True**   The bulk of the excess deaths suffered by cigarette smokers are from cardiovascular disease, of which coronary heart disease is the major component.

   D **False**   Depending on age groups the relative risk of lung cancer in a heavy cigarette smoker compared with a non-smoker can be 10–20 whereas that for coronary disease is 2–5. The reason why coronary disease is more important in absolute terms is because the risk of lung cancer in a non-smoker is extremely small, whereas that of developing coronary disease is substantial.

   E **False**   Countries like Japan have very high cigarette consumptions but there appears to be little coronary disease. Cigarette smoking promotes coronary disease only where population lipid levels are high. The relationship to lung cancer and respiratory disease is much more widespread.

1.9 A **False**   This is one of the occupations with a low lung cancer risk, probably because smoking at work is prohibited.

   B **True**   In the Northern hemisphere the prevaling winds are from the West so that air pollution is concentrated in the East End of major cities. This has interrelated effects, one being that any atmospheric contribution to lung disease is concentrated there (now diminished by Clean Air Acts), the second being that professional and administrative classes live in the West and semi and unskilled workers, who smoke more, live in the East.

   C **True**   Asbestos not only causes a rare tumour, mesothelioma, which is more specific for asbestos exposure, but also causes bronchial carcinoma, both in smokers and non-smokers. Smokers are at especially high risk.

   D **True**   There is a recognized occupational association between handling arsenicals and lung cancer. It is also a complication of the medicinal use of arsenic compounds.

   E **False**   Not recognized as an association. Mineral mines involving radioactive ores are a recognized hazard; radioactive gases are released. Salt mining does not have that association.

1.10 A **False** Standardized mortality ratios for doctors for cirrhosis of the liver are several times higher than the average for all occupied men and that for all professional men.

B **True** Britain used to have very low rates by international standards but the situation is changing and rates have risen considerably since World War II.

C **True** Rates are high in journalists, publicans and hotel keepers, in public relations and in show business, related to occupational exposure to heavy drinking.

D **True** There is a good correlation between the proportion of the population who drink heavily and develop alcohol related diseases, and the mean consumption of the whole population.

E **False** There is a correlation between the cost of alcohol in real terms and consumption. Cost in real terms in Britain has declined at the same time that consumption has gone up, as have alcohol related diseases and the same phenomenon has been demonstrated in other countries.

1.11 A **False** The disease reached a peak with the Great Depression of the 1930s when many children were malnourished. Rearmament and fuller employment were already improving nutrition before systematic attempts were made through fortified margarine, cod-liver oil and malt. Food rationing, although associated with shortages, was designed to ensure adequate nutrition, particularly for growing children.

B **True** Rickets re-emerged as a problem, of Asian immigrant families, in Britain in the 1950s and 1960s. Diet, racial pigmentation and avoidance of sunshine could all contribute.

C **False** Peak incidence clinically and biochemically occurs at times of minimum sunlight in the winter.

D **True** Certain substances in the diet, such as phytates, contained in chapatis, may inhibit the absorption of vitamin D even when it is present in small but potentially adequate quantities.

E **True** Lack of sunlight from air pollution and a high latitude contributed.

1.12 A **False**   One of the problems in the epidemiology of diabetes is in defining what diabetes is, by deciding on the cutting point in terms of a fasting, random or post glucose load blood sugar.

B **True**   As the population ages, new cases of diabetes occur, while most established cases remain, so that the prevalence in each age group is greater than in the previous one.

C **True**   The debate about whether obsessional blood sugar control prevents diabetic complications continues, but most patients' blood sugar control is less than perfect and the disease is associated with a reduced life expectancy.

D **False**   The number of diabetics who die from specific complications, such as hypoglycaemia or diabetic coma or renal complications, is small compared with those who develop cardiovascular disease and die from it, and in whom diabetes may not even be recorded on the death certificate.

E **False**   Incidence may be increased in industrialized sedentary populations, but it is found in many different Third World races and cultures.

1.13 A **False**   Morbidity data is collected on discharge when all investigations have been completed and a diagnosis made. Admission diagnoses are often different from discharge diagnoses, so details are collected on discharge. Some psychiatric hospitals do collect information on admission as well as discharge, because of the longer periods of hospitalization involved.

B **False**   Very little information is collected on out-patients in the UK other than in a few ad hoc projects.

C **False**   Again, other than for a few research projects, no details are collected on general practitioner consultations.

D **True**   Registration of new cancers is carried out throughout the UK by cancer registries and provides a unique source of information on cancer incidence.

E **True**   The General Household Survey contains questions on illness, although the exact questions asked vary from time to time.

1.14 A **False**   The World Health Organization (WHO) headquarters are in Geneva, Switzerland and there are a number of regional offices throughout the world.

B **True**   The funding of WHO is along similar lines to that of the UN; WHO was set up along with it.

C **True**   One of the major achievements of WHO was to co-ordinate the programmes which succeeded in eradicating smallpox.

D **False**   WHO produces a large number of publications including those on world health statistics, a weekly Epidemiological Record and journals such as the Bulletin of WHO, the WHO Chronicle and the Technical Report Series.

E **False**   WHO is concerned with all health matters and both communicable and non-communicable diseases.

1.15 A **False**   Social Work Departments are the responsibility of local government.

B **True**   Primary health care is provided by the local health authority.

C **False**   Again, this is the responsibility of local government and before the 1974 reorganization was part of the Medical Officer of Health organization. The health authority liaises with the local authority through the 'Proper Officer' or community medicine specialist for infectious diseases.

D **False**   These are quite separate from the health authorities.

E **True**   Community medical, nursing and dental services are all the responsibility of the health authorities.

1.16 A **True**   Around 70% of the expenditure in the NHS is on staff salaries. Although building and equipment costs in the health service are considerable, the majority of spending is on staff.

B **False**   The salaries of doctors are higher than most other employees in the health service but compared to other groups such as nurses their numbers are quite small. Most of the NHS salary bill goes to pay nurses.

C **True**   The expenditure on hospitals is much larger than that for community or primary care services.

D **True**   Acute services require expensive equipment and high staffing rates and take up more of the NHS resources than long-term care.

E **False**   All new capital developments in the NHS have revenue consequences and it is important to estimate these at the planning stage.

1.17 A **True** Each health authority has its own information service to provide the data required to evaluate and plan health services.

B **True** Claims for sickness benefit can be used to monitor morbidity but the diagnostic criteria are not very strict and the information is often spurious. Also, it is only for sickness absence of 7 days or longer.

C **True** Bed usage is a major part of information collected by health authorities in an attempt to monitor the efficiency of different wards.

D **True** The planning of health services is dependent on information collected on hospital bed usage, and demand for services. This information is used to predict future requirements.

E **True** Cancer registries are concerned with collecting information on all newly diagnosed cancers and these data are used to calculate incidence rates.

1.18 A **False** Disease notification is only of limited value and is dependent on doctors notifying health authorities. In practice, notification by doctors is variable and inconsistent.

B **False** Notification is controlled by legislation in individual countries and varies between countries and from time to time. Even within countries there may be variations in which diseases are notifiable.

C **True** Cholera is subject to the International Health Regulations, and along with plague and yellow fever is a quarantinable disease.

D **True** In several countries, including the UK, payments are made to doctors for notifying infectious diseases. Rewards were offered to the general public for reporting cases of smallpox during the WHO programme to eradicate the disease.

E **False** Notification of infectious disease is usually based on the reporting of syndromes, with no laboratory confirmation of infection.

1.19 A **True**   Pneumonia is the most common serious complication of measles infection and can be fatal in small children. Encephalitis may also cause death but is less common.

B **True**   Measles infection in malnourished children has a fatality rate of around 10%.

C **False**   The number of cases of measles infection in the USA has been reduced dramatically to only a few as the result of compulsory immunization. A valid certificate of measles immunization is required for school entry in the USA. An immunization rate of over 90% is required to prevent outbreaks.

D **False**   Measles vaccine is given in the second year of life. Earlier there may be persistent maternal antibody which prevents the development of immunity.

E **True**   A single dose of measles vaccine has a very high sero-conversion rate and the immunity derived is long lasting.

1.20 A **False**   Malaria prophylaxis is not 100% effective. It should not be assumed that a person who has taken prophylaxis cannot develop malaria.

B **False**   Pregnancy is not a contra-indication to malarial prophylaxis since the risks associated with malaria infection are greater than the risks of prophylaxis. Some prophylactic drugs such as sulfadoxine (Fansidar) are not recommended during pregnancy.

C **True**   Chloroquine resistant malaria is widespread throughout SE Asia, South America and East Africa.

D **True**   It is important that malaria prophylaxis in travellers is continued for one month after leaving the malarial area.

E **True**   In most cases of misdiagnosis of malaria, even if patients do not offer the information on foreign travel, medical practitioners have been considered negligent.

1.21 A False   Knowledge and behaviour are not closely related since behaviour is affected by attitudes, beliefs and peer group pressure.

B False   Few schools have courses specifically aimed at health education. Education for health may of course be taught as part of other subjects.

C False   Health education given by a doctor is effective as he/she is considered a credible source and has ready access to patients who may be in a receptive frame of mind.

D True   Most health authorities have centres or departments of health education run by health education officers.

E True   Health education is usually aimed at changing behaviour which will then affect health so there is a lag phase before any beneficial influence is seen.

1.22 A True   Houses suitable for habitation under the Housing Act are only required to meet tolerable standards.

B False   To meet tolerable standards a house should have an adequate supply of wholesome water and a sink supplying both hot and cold water.

C True   More than two persons per room would legally be overcrowding and thus not adequate housing.

D False   For tolerable housing standards a water closet should be available within the building, for exclusive use of the occupants.

E False   Housing is the responsibility of local government and inspections are carried out on its behalf.

Paper Two — Questions

2.1 A cohort (longitudinal) study differs from a case-control study in that
- A results are obtained less rapidly
- B it is only practicable for common diseases
- C it is possible to calculate relative risk
- D it is possible to measure incidence rates
- E risk factor assessment is more prone to bias

2.2 An epidemiological rate is described as crude if
- A it fails to observe the decencies of separating different age groups
- B it is given as per thousand instead of per hundred thousand
- C it is given to only two significant figures
- D it covers five years rather than one
- E it is based on an intercensal population estimate rather than a census figure

2.3 In randomized controlled trials
- A the patients recruited must be suitable for any of the treatments
- B treatments are allocated randomly to patients
- C patients are allocated randomly to treatments
- D assessment is always carried out by 'blinded' observers
- E a non-significant result in a trial means that the treatment is ineffective

2.4   Heavy cigarette smoking is associated with an excess mortality from cirrhosis of the liver. This implies that

A   there is a toxic effect of tobacco smoke on the liver
B   patients with any evidence of liver disease should not smoke
C   there could be an increased incidence of cirrhosis in cigarette smokers or diminished survival in those with cirrhosis, or both
D   malignant secondary deposits in the liver are being misdiagnosed as cirrhosis
E   in looking for evidence of causation it would be advisable to ensure that the heavy smoking preceded the onset of the cirrhosis

2.5   In population screening

A   the higher the sensitivity of a test, the smaller the proportion of false negatives
B   for tests of equal sensitivity, the lower the specificity, the lower the positive predictive value of the test
C   the higher the sensitivity of a test is set, the lower the specificity will be
D   the higher the sensitivity, the higher the measured prevalence rate of the disease
E   low repeatability does not imply a poor validity

2.6   The reported prevalence rate of a disease will increase (all else being constant) if

A   the incidence rate rises
B   survival time increases
C   recovery is delayed
D   diagnostic tests become more specific
E   the population in which it is measured increases

2.7   Coronary heart disease death rates

A   peak in middle age
B   are greater than those for breast cancer in women aged 35–54
C   result in the death of 10% of men by the age of 65 in high incidence countries such as Britain
D   are increasing in all Western countries
E   show the best correlation internationally with cigarette consumption

2.8   Serum cholesterol as a risk factor for coronary heart disease

A   is mostly explained by the presence of the gene for familial hypercholesterolaemia

B   is more specific for coronary disease than cigarette smoking and blood pressure

C   loses its power in older age groups

D   shows a gradient of increasing risk from low to high levels

E   identifies the 10% of middle-aged men who will develop coronary disease over the next 10 years

2.9   Regular cigarette smoking is associated with an increased risk of

A   lower limb amputation

B   death from paralysis agitans (Parkinson's disease)

C   lymphadenoma (Hodgkin's disease)

D   carcinoma of the bladder

E   bearing low birth-weight infants

2.10   Risk factors for carcinoma of the uterine cervix include

A   multiple marriages

B   being a nun

C   having a husband whose job takes him away from home a lot

D   late marriage

E   being an orthodox Jewess

2.11   Malignant melanoma rates are higher in

A   dark than in light skinned persons

B   Britain than in Australia

C   women than in men

D   unskilled workers than in professional workers

E   those exposed to fluorescent light during the working day

2.12   Duodenal ulcer

A   deaths are now commoner in the business and professional classes than in manual labourers

B   is declining as a cause of hospital admission

C   recurrence and healing are unaffected by cigarette smoking

D   incidence is equally common in men and women

E   natural history is revealed by mortality statistics

2.13   Care of the elderly

A   in residential homes is the responsibility of the health authority

B   at home for medical needs is the responsibility of the general practitioner

C   chronic sick at home in the UK is now uncommon

D   is now a decreasing problem in the UK

E   in sheltered housing is the responsibility of the local health authority

2.14   The allocation of resources to health authorities

A   is on the basis of population size alone
B   comes largely from National Insurance contributions
C   is distributed on an annual basis
D   is paid in part by local rates
E   is on a revenue and capital basis

2.15   Complaints about the health service can be investigated by

A   the Health Service Commissioner
B   the local health authority
C   the local government authority
D   the Community Health Councils
E   the Health Inspector

2.16   Expenditure in the NHS

A   on administration accounts for 20% of the total expenditure
B   on the elderly and children can be calculated using programme budgeting
C   is not greatly affected by wage rises
D   on preventative services is a considerable proportion of total expenditure
E   on residential homes for the elderly has greatly increased over the last 10 years

2.17   The NHS in the UK routinely

A   examines children when leaving school
B   requires all terminations of pregnancy to be notified within 7 days
C   screens all women over 20 years annually by cervical smears
D   screens contacts of pulmonary tuberculosis
E   provides family planning services free of charge

2.18   Paralytic poliomyelitis

A   virus is mainly spread by the faecal-oral route
B   can be caused by the oral polio vaccine
C   virus has two serotypes
D   occurs now in developing countries only
E   prevalence in developing countries can be estimated by lameness surveys

2.19 Healthy carrier

  A states lasting for more than a year are rare following Salmonella infections
  B states can occur in individuals with no clinical symptoms
  C individuals with *Salmonella typhi* can sometimes be corrected by appendicectomy
  D individuals with nasal meningococci should be treated with penicillin
  E individuals with *Salmonella typhi* may excrete the organism intermittently for the rest of their lives

2.20 Acquired immune deficiency syndrome

  A only affects men
  B is unknown before the age of 10 years
  C is characterized by a deficiency in humoral immunity
  D patients usually succumb to sarcoma or infection
  E was first reported in the UK in 1971

2.21 Air pollution

  A with lead varies with traffic density
  B from solids has health effects which are dependent on particle size
  C control has largely been through legislation
  D with sulphur dioxide is easily controlled because of its distinctive colour
  E with particulate matter can be controlled by electrostatic precipitation (ESP)

2.22 The Health and Safety Executive

  A has responsibility for investigating accidents at the workplace
  B is part of the Department of Health and Social Security (DHSS)
  C has no legal powers
  D is responsible for controlling under age working
  E was set up in 1974

Paper Two — Answers

2.1 A **True**   A case-control study starts with the cases: in a cohort study you must follow their occurrence in previously healthy people.

B **True**   A case-control study is the only practicable study for rare diseases, as cases can be taken from a population of millions, whereas the costs of cross-sectional and cohort studies are related to the number of healthy people that need to be studied to produce each case. A one per hundred prevalence or annual incidence rate can be studied, whereas one per thousand or ten thousand may not be cost-effective.

C **False**   Relative risk can be estimated in both.

D **True**   If you start with cases you cannot estimate the rate at which they are occurring: starting with a disease-free cohort you can.

E **False**   In a cohort study, risk factors are measured before the disease appears so the observer is blinded. In a case-control study, it is all too easy for the assessor to know or guess which are cases and which controls and to introduce bias in assessment of causal factors.

2.2 A **True** Crude rates are those that have not been broken down by age (and occasionally not by sex either), such as the all causes mortality rate for a total population, (total number of deaths/mid-year population) × 1000.

B **False** Crude rates are often given as rate per thousand but this is not invariable and not all rates per thousand are crude. Other bases are per 100 000, per million, etc.

C **False** Crude has a specific meaning; see A.

D **False** Crude has a specific meaning; see A.

E **False** Annual mortality rates are based on mid-year population estimates and this is true even for census years, as the census day is usually in April and not June 30th. Census figures may be used for five year cumulated rates, as for example in the Registrar General's reports on occupational mortality. Whether the denominator is an estimate, or derived more directly, does not determine whether a rate is considered crude.

2.3 A **True** The suitability of patients for the treatments is assessed before randomization. Patients who are unsuitable for one or more cannot be randomized and they should not be included in the trial.

B **True** Either the treatment or the patients are allocated and the effect is the same.

C **True** Either the treatments are randomly allocated to the patients or the patients are randomly allocated to the treatments and the effects are the same.

D **False** A trial in which patients and observers are blinded is called a 'double-blind' trial. Often trials are both randomized and double-blind but these are separate characteristics, and for some trials (such as those of surgery versus no surgery) it is possible to randomize treatment without being able, necessarily, to blind the observers. In such cases extreme efforts are needed to minimize the potential for observer bias.

E **False** The correct interpretation would be that within the limitations of the size of the study there is no definite evidence of advantage to either treatment. The study may have been too small to demonstrate a modest benefit (so called Type 2 error). Some trials compare two or more active drugs with each other so it is also possible that both treatments are equally effective.

2.4 A **False**   Association does not always mean causation. In this case the effect is believed to be mediated by the strong association between heavy alcohol consumption and heavy cigarette smoking.

B **False**   No-one should smoke, but this evidence of association is not good enough in itself to suggest, as is implied, that the prognosis of the liver disease would be affected by cessation.

C **True**   An increase in mortality might be associated with one or both of these mechanisms, in this case perhaps both.

D **False**   This is a possible explanation, but does not follow necessarily from the observed association.

E **True**   Cigarette smoking is not a particularly good example, as it is a habit acquired in youth, but it is always important to check whether an association might be an effect of the disease and not a cause. Patients ill with cirrhosis might conceivably smoke more after developing the disease but not beforehand.

2.5 A **True**   The sensitivity of the test is the proportion of true positives correctly identified, so that the higher it is, the lower the number of false negatives.

B **True**   A low specificity will result in a large number of false positive diagnoses resulting in a dilution of true positives. Of those screened positive a low proportion will be true cases so that the positive predictive value of the test will be low, however sensitive it is.

C **True**   You cannot get something for nothing. As one increases, the other decreases. It is unlikely that tests will have perfect sensitivity and specificity unless they are the 'gold standard' for diagnosis, but these are usually too expensive to use for population screening. In any given test it is usually necessary to set a cutting point. In such a case it is inevitable that as the threshold for screening positive is changed, sensitivity and specificity will increase or decrease in opposite directions.

D **True**   More true cases will be correctly identified. In addition specificity will probably fall (see C) so more false positives will appear; the proportion of any sort of positive in the population will therefore increase.

E **False**   Repeatability means that the test will tend to produce the same result when repeated, whereas validity means that it is measuring what it purports to measure. A test of low repeatability cannot have a high validity as it cannot be right consistently if it gives inconsistent answers.

2.6 A **True**   If all other factors are constant, the greater the rate at which new cases appear, the greater the proportion of the population that will have the disease at any one time.

B **True**   The longer the average duration of the illness, the higher the proportion of the population affected at any one time.

C **True**   Same argument as in B. Prevalence can be reduced by cure or death.

D **False**   If the diagnostic tests are more specific they will be less prone to produce false positives. The measured and reported prevalence rate for the condition will therefore decline. As tests become more specific there may also be a decline in sensitivity as well. Although this is not always true, it would also contribute to an apparent decline.

E **False**   Use of a disease rate automatically compensates for changes in the population denominator so there should be no necessary change.

2.7 A **False**   This is a common clinical fallacy. In successive age groups numbers increase and then fall again but when these numbers are related to the diminishing age specific population, as is done in disease rates, it can be seen that mortality rates go on increasing throughout the age range.

B **False**   The common statement that coronary disease is the major cause of death in middle age is true for men (and for both sexes considered together, as male death rates are so much higher) but not true for women considered alone. In women cancer is a greater cause of death in middle age, and breast cancer is a bigger hazard than coronary disease.

C **True**   This single disease, at current rates, will cause the death of one man in ten before age 65.

D **False**   There is considerable variation between one country and another. Rates are falling in the US and Australia and also in Belgium; they may be beginning to fall in the UK and they are still rising in some other countries.

E **False**   International differences in coronary heart disease mortality are poorly explained by cigarette consumption. For example, Japan has low coronary rates, as does France, but smoking rates are high.

2.8 A **False**   The gene frequency of familial hypercholesterolaemia is at most 1 in 300 of the population while coronary disease and raised serum cholesterol are very much commoner. A very small percentage of coronary disease and of high cholesterol readings are therefore attributable to this gene.

B **True**   Serum cholesterol is one of the three major risk factors for coronary disease, and possibly the fundamental one, as it explains international differences better than do smoking and blood pressure. However, smoking and blood pressure predict major diseases other than coronary disease, whereas serum cholesterol does not; it is specific for coronary disease.

C **True**   Serum cholesterol is a good predictor in young men but over the age of 60 it loses most of its power.

D **True**   There is a gradient of risk across the whole range of cholesterol readings, although the gradient rises more sharply at higher levels. There is therefore no threshold below which all readings have the same significance.

E **False**   Neither serum cholesterol nor any of the other risk factors, alone or in combination, can predict perfectly who will and who will not develop coronary disease within a certain period. It will discriminate good and bad risk groups, but within these groups most individuals will remain well.

2.9 A **True**   It is the major risk-factor both for the development and the progression to gangrene of peripheral vascular disease, leading to amputation. Road accidents are also commoner in smokers.

B **False**   There is a lower than expected death rate from this disease in cigarette smokers, one of the very few medically authenticated benefits.

C **False**   No association.

D **True**   This association has been consistently demonstrated and a possible mechanism could exist through urinary concentration of inhaled carcinogens.

E **True**   This has been demonstrated in a number of studies, some of which have gone on to suggest that the stunting of growth persists.

2.10 A True   Early onset of sexual activity, exposure to many partners, or a partner who is promiscuous, appear to increase the risk.

  B False   Nuns who have never been married are said to be free of the disease, an observation first made about 200 years ago.

  C True   There are high rates in wives of seamen and transport workers.

  D False   Late marriage correlates with late onset of sexual activity.

  E False   Studies in the USA and Israel suggested that carcinoma of the cervix was rare in orthodox Jewish families and a variety of explanations have been advanced, including the effects of circumcision, and of the customary abstinence from sexual intercourse for a period after menstruation ceases.

2.11 A False   Paradoxically, the presence of melanin in the skin appears to protect against the development of melanoma.

  B False   Rates are higher in white skinned populations nearer the equator, possibly because skin damage from sunlight is greater.

  C True   Women have higher rates than men.

  D False   One of the few tumours with a negative social class gradient, that is, it is commoner in professional and administrative groups.

  E True   Several case-control studies suggest that occupational exposure to fluorescent light is a risk factor, and one even suggests that it is fluorescent lights without diffusers that are at fault. The association puzzles physicists who think the energy level at different wavelengths makes the association implausible.

2.12 A **False**   When the disease was increasing in incidence it appeared commoner in the upper social classes while gastric ulcers showed the opposite distribution. A generation later it appears that both gastric and duodenal ulcers are behaving in the same way.

   B **True**   Both admissions for severe ulcer symptoms and for complications such as bleeding and perforation are declining.

   C **False**   It is claimed that continuation of smoking affects ulcer healing and recurrence adversely.

   D **False**   Duodenal ulcers are commoner in men.

   E **False**   Natural history implies course and prognosis. Death certificates record only the alleged disease held responsible for the subject's death, so only those ulcers recognized as contributing to death will appear and no others.

2.13 A **False**   Residential homes are run by the Social Work Departments of the local government and not by the health authority.

   B **True**   General practitioners provide medical care for the elderly at home but may be assisted by domiciliary assessment by geriatricians.

   C **False**   Although a large number of the elderly chronic sick are in hospitals and nursing homes, the majority are cared for in their own homes.

   D **False**   The proportion of the population over 75 years of age is still increasing, that over 85 years of age even more so.

   E **False**   Sheltered housing is run by the housing departments of local government authorities and not by the health authorities.

2.14 A **False**   Many factors are taken into consideration in deciding the resource allocation to health authorities under the RAWP (Resource Allocation Working Party) in England and Wales, and SHARE (Scottish Health Authorities Revenue Equalization) in Scotland.

   B **False**   National Insurance contributions are only a small fraction of the source of NHS funding; the majority comes from central taxation.

   C **True**   The resource allocation is carried out annually over the financial year commencing April 1st.

   D **False**   Local rates are not used to fund the health service.

   E **True**   Revenue (running costs) expenditure and capital expenditure are both taken into account in resource allocation.

2.15 A **True**   The Health Service Commissioner is responsible for investigating complaints by individuals about the health service.

B **True**   Health authorities have their own procedures for investigating any complaints about their service or staff.

C **False**   Local government has no role in investigating NHS complaints.

D **True**   The complaints dealt with by the Community Health Councils are more general in nature and not the complaints of an individual.

E **False**   Health inspection work is carried out by Environmental Health Departments and has nothing to do with NHS complaints.

2.16 A **False**   Expenditure on administration in the NHS is around 5% of the total expenditure. Many large industries have administration costs of around 15%.

B **True**   Programme budgeting is a method of overviewing the expenditure in the Health Service. It considers expenditure in terms of input to particular client groups, e.g. the elderly, disease groups, or geographical areas.

C **False**   The expenditure on wages and salaries in the NHS is around 70% of the total expenditure so any change in salaries will have a great effect on expenditure.

D **False**   The expenditure on preventative services and health education is a negligible part of health service expenditure.

E **False**   Residential homes for care of the elderly are provided through local government authorities and not by the health service.

2.17 A **True**   All children are routinely examined in the UK, at school entry and when leaving school, by a clinical medical officer.

B **True**   There is a statutory requirement for the doctor performing a termination of pregnancy to notify the fact within 7 days.

C **False**   Cervical smears are usually performed every 3–5 years on women over the age of 35 years. They are also taken at post-natal examinations.

D **True**   Contacts of pulmonary tuberculosis at home and at work are followed up and screened by chest x-ray.

E **True**   All family planning services in the UK are provided free of charge, including prescriptions for the contraceptive pill.

2.18 A **True** The poliovirus is a member of the enterovirus group and is primarily a gastrointestinal infection. The nervous system is involved secondarily, and in only a minority of poliovirus infections.

B **True** The live oral vaccine (Sabin) regains virulence by successive infections and may result in paralytic disease. This affects the unimmunized contacts of recently vaccinated children, especially unprotected parents of recently immunized children.

C **False** The virus has three serotypes: 1, 2 and 3. This is the rationale for giving a three dose course of vaccine, since only one serotype may take with a single dose of vaccine. The vaccine contains all three serotypes.

D **False** Most developed countries have a few sporadic cases of paralytic poliomyelitis each year. There have also been recent outbreaks in the Netherlands, USA and Canada.

E **True** In countries where there is no good notification system or laboratory facilities, surveys of lameness are frequently used to assess the magnitude of the problem in the community.

2.19 A **True** Temporary carrier states after a Salmonella infection occasionally continue for a few months, but chronic carrier states for longer than one year are very uncommon.

B **True** By definition, healthy carriers of an infectious agent should have no symptoms or signs of infection, other than carriage of the organism.

C **False** Bacilli may persist in the gall bladder and pass intermittently in the stools and for this reason cholecystectomy is sometimes performed, but not appendicectomy.

D **False** Carriage rates of nasal meningococci may be as high as 25% in a community with no evidence of meningitis so little is gained by attempting treatment. Meningococci are not fully eradicated from the oro-nasopharynx by penicillin; sulphonamides are more effective.

E **True** Although chronic carriage is uncommon, it can be life long.

2.20 A **False**   While many cases are in male homosexuals, the syndrome has been diagnosed in prostitutes, in drug addicts who share needles and in recipients of pooled clotting factors of both sexes.

B **False**   There is a growing number of pre-school children in whom the syndrome has been diagnosed.

C **False**   The main deficiency is in cellular and not humoral immunity.

D **True**   The commonest causes of death in patients with this syndrome are Kaposi's sarcoma and opportunistic infections, especially Pneumocystis carinii pneumonia.

E **False**   The first formal report of the syndrome in the UK was in 1981.

2.21 A **True**   The concentration of lead in air varies with traffic density, although traffic speed and weather conditions influence the levels of lead.

B **True**   The smaller size particles are inhaled and can pass through the bronchial tree and are associated with greater morbidity.

C **True**   Legislation, in a number of statutes over the years, has had the most effect on air pollution control.

D **False**   Sulphur dioxide is colourless and most control measures of pollution are based on coloured smoke. Large emissions of sulphur dioxide high in the atmosphere have contributed to the acid rain phenomenon.

E **True**   Electrostatic precipitation is commonly used to remove particulate matter from emissions, before these are discharged into the atmosphere.

2.22 A **True**   An important function is the investigation of industrial accidents and dangerous practices.

B **False**   The Health and Safety Executive is administered by the Department of Employment and has its own medical arm, the Employment Medical Advisory Service (EMAS).

C **False**   The Health and Safety Executive has wide powers to enforce the regulations of the various employment acts.

D **True**   This is part of the Executive's functions, along with control of the hours of employment.

E **True**   The Executive and Commission were set up in 1974 following the passing by parliament of the Health and Safety at Work Act, 1974.

Paper Three — Questions

3.1 Infant mortality rate
A is calculated using census data
B is the sum of the perinatal and post-neonatal rates
C is higher in girl infants
D is lower in breast fed babies
E shows no social class gradient under the Welfare State

3.2 Medical certificates of cause of death
A are issued by the same person as the official death certificate
B can only be issued by a medical practitioner (or a coroner)
C can be issued when death appears to be imminent
D are used to generate national statistics on age, sex and cause-specific mortality
E are based on an international design agreed through WHO

3.3 A cross-sectional study differs from a cohort (longitudinal) study in that
A it is not done on a defined population
B risk-factors are ascertained at the same time as the disease
C it is usually cheaper
D relative risks cannot be calculated, even with retrospective risk factor data
E it cannot be used to measure incidence rates

3.4 Since 1968 the crude mortality rate for a chronic disease has increased. Possible explanations are that
A there has been a true increase in the age- and sex-specific incidence rates
B there has been no change in incidence but a greater tendency to record the diagnosis at death certification
C age-specific mortality rates have remained static
D case fatality has increased
E there has been a drift into other diagnostic categories

3.5   When taking blood pressure with a standard mercury sphygmomanometer

A   repeated observations by the same observer will not remove observer bias
B   observers of the same sex as the subject produce higher readings
C   digit preference is an indicator of the degree of imprecision
D   the normal blood pressure is 120/80 mmHg
E   patients characterized as having extreme readings on one occasion are likely to be less extreme when the reading is repeated

3.6   The prevalence rate of a disease could be estimated from

A   the percentage of hospital discharges with that diagnosis
B   a cross-sectional survey
C   the ratio of cases to controls in a case-control study
D   a survey of outpatients attending a general clinic
E   the flagging of cases in a general practice with an age/sex register

3.7   The following are significant risk-factors for coronary heart disease

A   smoking a pipe
B   adding sugar to tea or coffee
C   a raised systolic blood pressure
D   a professional life
E   low serum levels of high density lipoprotein cholesterol

3.8   Mild hypertension

A   is diagnosable from a single blood-pressure reading
B   is a major risk factor for coronary heart disease
C   is prognostically more serious in men than women
D   is usually associated with typical symptoms
E   treatment, even with single drugs, often produces side effects

3.9   Chronic obstructive airways disease

A   prevention has been attempted by national legislation
B   prevalence can be assessed by questionnaires
C   occurs uniformly across the social classes
D   is diminishing as a cause of death in Britain
E   is a notifiable industrial disease

3.10 Carcinoma of the breast
A is prevented by breast feeding
B is associated with obesity in post-menopausal women
C is commoner in single than in married women
D is declining as a cause of death in women in Britain
E deaths all occur within five years of onset

3.11 Risk-factors for diabetes mellitus include
A female sex
B obesity
C known genetic markers
D major population lifestyle changes
E virus infection in the case of maturity onset, non insulin dependent diabetes

3.12 Large bowel cancer
A is commoner in countries with a rice and fish diet
B prognosis is related to histological staging
C prognosis is influenced by risk of recurrent primary tumours
D is considerably commoner in women than men
E risk is increased in cigarette smokers

3.13 Environmental Health Departments
A are responsible to local government
B carry out duties under the Health and Safety at Work Act
C have to pay the wages of people kept off work because they may endanger public health
D carry out regular inspections of restaurants
E are run by the Medical Officer of Health

3.14 Demand for health care
A is what the population needs
B is relatively simple to assess
C is adequately met by the NHS
D varies between social classes
E is greatest in developing countries

3.15 Management in the NHS
A is responsible for setting objectives for health care
B requires to work closely with health service trade unions
C needs to collect information on health service activities
D faces major problems of inertia in the service
E can be efficient without being effective

3.16 Bed occupancy

A   is highest in acute wards
B   is generally low in long-stay units
C   is a method of assessing effectiveness in the health service
D   is calculated from the daily occupied beds and the number of beds available
E   varies between different specialities

3.17 The health visitor is

A   employed by the local government authority
B   largely concerned with prevention
C   a trained nurse
D   concerned with the health of children under five years old
E   supervised by a general practitioner

3.18 Vaccines

A   for mumps are used in many countries
B   should be safer than therapies
C   are never effective after exposure to the infectious agent
D   were largely responsible for the decline in mortality from infectious diseases in developed countries
E   against measles and rubella are live attenuated viruses

3.19 Tuberculosis

A   is usually a primary infection in the elderly
B   can usually be prevented by BCG alone
C   is still a major cause of premature death in most developing countries
D   has been predominantly controlled in developed countries by pasteurization of milk
E   vaccine — BCG — may also prevent leprosy

3.20 Cyclical patterns of infection

A   are typical of measles
B   in the descending phase are the result of a fall in the number of susceptible individuals
C   decrease in frequency in the more densely populated areas
D   can be simulated by mathematical models
E   reflect the rise and fall in the proportion of immune individuals in a community

3.21 Air pollution

A   has an effect only in the immediate neighbourhood of the source
B   is rapidly cleared by temperature inversions
C   is associated with increased mortality from all causes and not just respiratory diseases
D   and mist result in smog
E   is more important in the causation of lung cancer than tobacco smoking

3.22 The most important factor in the prevention of

A   dental caries is regular teeth brushing
B   lung cancer is stopping cigarette smoking
C   stroke is control of blood pressure
D   cholera is immunization with the cholera vaccine
E   coronary heart disease is taking active exercise

Paper Three — Answers

3.1 A **False**   Unlike many other mortality rates the infant mortality rate does not use census data, but the number of registered live births in the year.

     B **False**   Perinatal deaths include still-births, which form neither part of the numerator or the denominator for infant mortality rates, and they stop at one week whereas the post-neonatal period starts at 29 days.

     C **False**   Like mortality rates at all other ages, there is a considerably higher rate in males.

     D **True**   This seems to be generally true both in affluent and third world countries. Babies fed artificially are more prone to infection, particularly infantile diarrhoea.

     E **False**   Infant mortality rates have declined considerably since the World War II but social class gradients have been preserved.

3.2 A **False**   The medical certificate of cause of death is issued by a medical practitioner to the relative or informant, who takes it to the local Registrar of Births and Deaths, who uses this plus other information to generate the official death certificate. It is the latter which is the legal document, a copy of which is sent to the Registrar General's office.

B **True**   Certifying death, and prescribing and administering certain drugs, are some of the very few things specifically reserved by law to medical practitioners. The exception is in deaths referred to the coroner where he or she may certify the cause of death (usually from evidence produced by a pathologist), but the coroner may or may not be medically qualified.

C **False**   The medical certificate gives the option of the body being seen by the signing practitioner or by another practitioner. As it is used to provide a legal document showing that death has occurred it cannot be issued in anticipation.

D **True**   Death certificate data are cumulated centrally in the Registrar General's offices and collated with census data or intercensal estimates of the population at risk in order to generate death rates.

E **True**   The design of death certificates results from international agreements, which seek to standardize reporting of mortality statistics so that different countries can be compared.

3.3 A **False** The denominator for both cross-sectional (prevalence) and cohort (longitudinal) studies must be a defined population group. Many cohort studies start with a cross-sectional survey which then leads to the follow-up of incidence.

B **True** In a single cross-sectional study the prevalence cases of disease are identified at the same survey as the risk factors are looked at, whereas in a cohort study the risk factors are identified in advance of the incidence cases of the disease.

C **True** Most cohort studies incorporate an initial cross-sectional study and some (e.g. the Framingham study of coronary heart disease) include repeated re-examinations, each of which is equivalent in cost to a cross-sectional study. There is also the cost in cohort studies of tracing people for disease incidence. It is possible to envisage cohort studies with no screening and cheap follow-up however (e.g. flagging workers exposed to a toxic chemical for mortality follow-up).

D **False** Relative risk can be calculated from a cross-sectional study in which past history of risk-factors and prevalence cases of disease are identified.

E **True** Incidence is a measure of disease occurrence over time and therefore it cannot be measured in a cross-sectional study, which takes place at one time for any given individual. However, age-specific prevalence rates may be used to calculate incidence under special circumstances.

3.4 A **True** In the presence of an aging population an increase in age-specific rates will lead to an even larger increase in crude mortality rates.

B **True** Serious diagnoses such as cancer are often missing from death certificates or may not appear as the underlying cause of death. For example, a terminal pulmonary embolus or pneumonia may be coded as the underlying cause of death when the patient had carcinomatosis from a diagnosed primary.

C **True** There has been a substantial aging of the population, with a reduction in the proportion of young people, so that all-ages death rates can go up even when age-specific rates remain constant.

D **True** If the number of new cases is the same, but more are dying, then the mortality rate will be increased.

E **False** Mortality rates reflect what is diagnosed so that loss of potential diagnoses to other categories will lead to a decline.

3.5 A **True**   Repeated observations will lower the effect of random variation in the readings, but much of observer variation or bias is systematic, and will not be affected.

B **False**   Observers of the opposite sex (and different ethnic group) to the observer tend to obtain higher readings.

C **True**   Blood pressure is continuously distributed so that the different digits should be equally represented. Digit preference indicates that rounding up and down is occurring. In epidemiological studies even numbered digits are used. Clinicians tend to use 5s and 0s, some measure to the nearest 10, and 20s may figure disproportionately. Analysis reveals the imprecision.

D **False**   120/80 may have been a historical average for young people but it has little statistical or epidemiological basis and is unrepresentative of middle age where most readings are taken and 145/85 would be more typical. A range of normal is more useful than a single value. What is normal may not be desirable; the lower the individual's blood pressure the lower the cardiovascular risk. High average may be harmful and abnormally low beneficial. The word 'normal' has to be defined therefore.

E **True**   Among those with extreme readings will be those who have a less extreme reading on average but were picked out because they were at an extreme; their readings will be nearer their average on the next occasion. This phenomenon, called regression to the mean, is more of a problem with unstable factors such as blood pressure or serum cholesterol than with stable ones such as height.

3.6 A **False**   Hospital inpatients are a biased sample of the population. For this measure to work it would mean that the presence of the disease was completely unassociated with the reasons for admission, and that despite this fact it was always recorded at discharge, an inherently improbable combination.

  B **True**   In a cross-sectional survey of a defined population group the prevalence rate will be the proportion of subjects with the disease at the time they were surveyed.

  C **False**   The ratio of cases to controls is determined by the investigator and is usually a simple multiple. Case-control studies are often done on rare conditions whose prevalence rate in the community is one in tens of thousands.

  D **False**   The same objections apply here as to A. General hospital outpatients cannot be considered as a typical population sample and their reasons for attending the hospital clinic may bias their probability of suffering from the disease in question.

  E **True**   A complete record of all diagnosed cases in a practice, for a disease that always comes to medical attention, related to the at-risk population obtained from the age-sex register, would give the prevalence rate within that practice.

3.7 A **False**   Lifelong pipe smoking confers little added risk to that of being a non-smoker. Cigarette smokers who adopt a pipe or cigars tend to go on inhaling heavily, however, and this could be as dangerous.

  B **False**   Despite the common belief, sugar in itself is not considered to be atherogenic; as part of an excess calorie intake leading to obesity it could be, and a sweet tooth is often associated with cigarette smoking.

  C **True**   Above average levels of systolic or diastolic blood pressure are predictive of increased risk.

  D **False**   Professional workers have below average risk of coronary disease and there is little formal evidence that hard work is harmful, although some studies have suggested that subjects who set themselves multiple deadlines have more heart-attacks than those who take things less competitively.

  E **True**   High density lipoprotein cholesterol appears to be protective. It makes up a small proportion of the total circulating cholesterol concentration, levels of which in serum or plasma are positively associated with risk. Its importance may have been exaggerated in the 1970s.

3.8 A **False**   A single raised blood pressure reading is an indication to repeat the measurement. Because of the considerable within person variation, the diagnosis of mild hypertension should never be based on a single reading.

B **True**   The majority of coronary deaths that are attributable to raised blood pressure occur in those whose pressure is only mildly elevated.

C **True**   For the same level of blood pressure men run a much higher risk of coronary heart disease, which is the major hazard associated with mild hypertension; risk of stroke being much less.

D **False**   Most mild hypertension is asymptomatic although it is often first identified when patients attend complaining of indeterminate symptoms.

E **True**   The Medical Research Council mild hypertension trial showed that diuretics and beta blockers, thought to be comparatively free of side effects, when tested against placebo produced a high incidence of side effects which led to discontinuation of therapy.

3.9 A **True**   The clean-air acts of the 1950s and 1960s were designed to reduce the morbidity and mortality from chronic bronchitis and emphysema from atmospheric pollution.

B **True**   Symptom questionnaires, such as that for chronic bronchitis used in Medical Research Council surveys, have been used to compare the prevalence of disease in different population groups.

C **False**   There is a strongly positive social class gradient with a much higher prevalence in unskilled outdoor occupations than in indoor professional ones, although this association is now probably reinforced by class differences in cigarette smoking.

D **True**   There has been a decline as particulate air pollution has improved, and the amount of smoking and what is smoked has also changed.

E **False**   Although it may be commoner in certain occupations it is not specific enough to be notifiable, and is strongly related to non-occupational factors such as cigarette smoking and air pollution.

3.10 A False Childbearing at an early age appears protective, while breast feeding, although desirable on other grounds, does not appear to confer additional protection.

 B True An epidemiological observation which may be explained by the metabolism of oestrogens in fatty tissues.

 C True The exact opposite of carcinoma of the cervix, which never occurs in virgins, carcinoma of the breast (and the ovary) are commoner in old maids.

 D False Unfortunately breast cancer is a major and increasing cause of death in women.

 E False Breast cancers can be slow growing, and metastases can appear years after the patient is thought to have been cured.

3.11 A False Although this was commonly reported, systematic population surveys suggest that there is no difference between the sexes.

 B True There is a confirmed association between maturity onset diabetes and obesity.

 C True Genetic markers exist for both insulin dependent (certain HLA types) and non insulin dependent diabetes (chlorpropamide alcohol flushing).

 D True The incidence of diabetes rises rapidly in populations which are experiencing the transition from heavy physical activity and periods of hunger to mechanization, physical inactivity and steady food supplies.

 E False Viral infection with Coxsackie B4 may often precede insulin dependent diabetes occurring in childhood, but there is no such association recognized for non insulin dependent diabetes which, in any case, has a much less clear-cut onset.

3.12 A False Incidence is low in countries such as Japan with a rice and fish diet. Immigrants from Japan increase their risk as they adopt the North American diet.

 B True Prognosis is related to the degree of spread from the mucosa.

 C True This is one of the tumours where completely successful removal of the primary lesion still leaves the patient at considerably increased risk of further malignancy, unless the whole of the large bowel has been removed.

 D False The incidence is similar in men and women, although differences occur in different parts of the large bowel.

 E False Studies of cigarette smokers have not been consistent in showing an increased risk of large bowel cancer.

3.13 A **True**   Environmental Health Departments are part of the local government organization although health authorities provide medical advice.

B **True**   Part of the duties of Environmental Health Departments is to carry out inspections of smaller premises and work places.

C **True**   Wages are made up, including estimated overtime, by the Environmental Health Departments of individuals kept from work because they constitute a public health risk.

D **True**   Inspections of places where food handling is carried out are the responsibility of Environmental Health Departments.

E **False**   The Medical Officer of Health position now no longer exists. Before 1974, the work of the Environmental Health Departments was carried out by the Medical Officer of Health.

3.14 A **False**   Demand and need are quite separate concepts. Demand is what the community wants themselves, while need has to be determined by a third party.

B **True**   What a community demands is usually made clear whereas need is very difficult to assess objectively.

C **False**   Demand for health care is limitless and so can never be met by any health service.

D **True**   There is an important gradient in demand for health care by social class. In general the higher social classes demand health care more but need it less than lower social classes.

E **False**   The demand for health care is greatest in the countries with the most advanced health care systems. The need, however, for health care is greatest in developing countries.

3.15 A **True**   It is essential in management to be able to set objectives and plan a health service to meet these objectives. Without objectives the management process would be completely aimless.

B **True**   Management in modern society needs to work closely with unions and be in continual consultation with representatives of the work force. The NHS consults with many trade unions, including the doctors' union, the British Medical Association. Trade union representatives are also members of health authority boards and community health councils.

C **True**   The health service management needs to collect information, to assess its performance, and to see whether or not the objectives set are being met. Also it is necessary to identify new problem areas requiring attention.

D **True**   All large organization have an inbuilt resistance to change and the NHS is no exception. To progress, it is essential to overcome this inertia.

E **True**   Efficiency is concerned with achieving an end with the minimum of resources; effectiveness is concerned with whether this end attains the beneficial result for which it was designed (e.g. contrast the most efficient system of screening for hypertension with whether blood pressure screening effectively lowers stroke deaths).

3.16 A **False**   The occupancy in acute wards is usually lower because of the need to have free beds at any time to accept emergency admissions.

B **False**   The occupancy in long-stay wards usually approaches 100% as the turnover is slow and empty beds are quickly filled.

C **False**   Bed occupancy is a method of assessing the efficiency of bed use in a hospital but says nothing about effectiveness.

D **True**   Bed occupancy is calculated from the beds occupied each day as a percentage of the average number of beds available.

E **True**   There are large variations between specialities in bed occupancy. Paediatric and obstetric wards usually have low occupancy and geriatric wards usually have high occupancy.

3.17 A False   Health visitors are employed by the health authority. Prior to the 1974 NHS reorganization they were employed by the local government authority.

B True   Health visitors are concerned more with prevention than with the day to day care of patients.

C True   Health visiting is a part of the nursing profession. Health visitors are all trained nurses with obstetric experience and undergo one year of further training.

D True   A large part of the work of the health visitor is with children under five years old concerning feeding, immunization and development.

E False   Health visitors usually work alongside general practitioners but are professionals in their own right and not responsible to doctors.

3.18 A True   Mumps vaccine is now used in many developed countries including Scandanavia and the USA. The vaccine is usually given combined with measles and rubella vaccines in the second year of life.

B True   Vaccines are usually given to healthy individuals, so the safety standards must be much higher than those for therapeutic measures which are administered to individuals who have disease.

C False   Vaccines can be effective post exposure in diseases with long incubation periods. Rabies is a good example. The vaccine can stimulate protective immunity after exposure to the virus.

D False   The major decline in mortality from infectious diseases in developed countries occurred before the introduction of vaccines, and probably resulted from nutritional and socio-economic improvements.

E True   Rubella and measles vaccines are both live attenuated virus vaccines. This is important to remember when considering immunization of pregnant women and immune compromised patients.

3.19 A False   In the elderly, tuberculosis is usually a reactivation of an earlier focus of infection, which may occur in association with concurrent disease or steroid therapy.

B False   The effectiveness of BCG in preventing tuberculosis is very variable and is much less important than socio-economic improvements in preventing tuberculosis.

C True   Tuberculosis is still endemic in many developing countries and one of the major causes of death.

D False   Pasteurization of milk only controls milk borne infection and has no effect on the airborne droplet infection of Mycobacterium tuberculosis.

E True   Leprosy is also caused by a mycobacterium and there is a degree of cross-reaction. Trials have shown that BCG can prevent leprosy.

3.20 A True   Measles epidemics usually occur in two to three year cycles.

B True   During an epidemic, as more people become infected, the proportion susceptible falls and the epidemic wanes.

C False   In sparsely populated areas the number of person to person contacts are smaller and cycles of infection tend to be infrequent.

D True   Mathematical modelling of infectious disease patterns is commonly used to predict levels of immunity required to end epidemics in a population.

E True   The changes in the proportions of immune individuals result in the cyclic patterns of infection. Infection usually results in immunity while births and immigration introduce new susceptible people.

3.21 A **False** Air pollution has local and distant effects. The distant effects may involve whole continents and depend on weather conditions and the height of emissions into the atmosphere.

B **False** Temperature inversions prevent pollutants being dispersed by convection currents, thus increasing the concentration of the pollutants locally.

C **True** The effect of air pollution is seen in many causes of death other than respiratory diseases. People already disabled by disease are at increased risk of death in the presence of air pollution.

D **True** Air pollution and mist result in smog. This prevents sunshine penetrating to the ground so that more people light fires for warmth and increase the pollution. The London smogs of the early 1950s were associated with large increases in mortality.

E **False** The contribution of air pollution to the causation of lung cancer is small in comparison to the effect of smoking.

3.22 A **False** While brushing prevents gum disease, reduced dietary sugar and fluoride are more important in the prevention of caries.

B **True** Cigarette smoking is the most important cause of lung cancer and stopping (or never starting) reduces the risk of cancer.

C **True** Hypertension is the most important risk factor for stroke and its control is associated with reduced risk.

D **False** Cholera vaccine is only of limited value, much more important is adequate sewage disposal and a clean, safe, water supply.

E **False** The three most important risk factors for coronary heart disease are smoking, blood pressure and serum cholesterol level.

Paper Four — Questions

4.1 Relative risk

A for a risk-factor is usually the ratio of the risk of those with the factor and those without it

B is better than attributable risk for showing that a risk-factor is likely to be causally associated with a disease

C cannot be estimated from a case-control study

D unlike attributable risk, does not quantify risk in absolute terms

E can be low for a factor with a high attributable risk

4.2 A study showed that the majority of motor cyclists who were killed were males aged 17–20 years of age. This demonstrates that

A most motor cyclists are males aged 17–20

B it is safer to ride motor cycles when over this age

C it is safer to learn to ride motor cycles when over this age

D other road users persecute young male motor cyclists

E women motor cyclists are much safer than men

4.3 Epidemiology is

A concerned only with the study of infectious disease epidemics

B the only source of information on disease causation

C the study of the distribution and determinants of disease in human populations

D concerned with both common and rare diseases

E the study of the epidermis

4.4 Trends in standardized mortality rates for a disease over time may be seriously affected by

A the age and sex distribution of the population

B revision of the International Classification of Diseases

C changes in medico-legal practice

D fashions in diagnosis

E acceptability of vague or inadequate diagnoses

4.5 Epidemiological measures of disease frequency are interrelated so that

A if the incidence rate of a disease is increasing there will be an increase in the case fatality rate

B the prevalence rate will increase if average survival time increases

C unless rates are changing the mortality rate cannot be greater than the incidence rate

D the incidence rate is reduced by an increase in the recovery rate

E mortality and case fatality rates are equal

4.6 In a case-control study

A the number of controls need not equal the number of cases

B cases and controls should be matched for the risk factors under investigation

C relative risk can be calculated

D ascertainment of risk factors is retrospective

E rare diseases cannot be investigated

4.7 In the so called 'prudent diet' to lower coronary risk

A low cholesterol and cholesterol lowering are the same

B all animal fats should be avoided and all vegetable fats are good

C vegetables and fruit should be avoided because they contain sugar

D the majority of the population can lower serum cholesterol by diet

E no large randomized controlled trial has shown that diet alone reduces coronary risk

4.8 Stroke

A death rates are very similar in middle-aged men and women

B risk is related more strongly to blood pressure than anything else

C is common in many countries where coronary disease is rare

D survivors usually die from a recurrent stroke

E most often leaves sequelae that would be detectable in a survey

4.9 Death rates from accidents

A are higher in males than females at all ages

B are the major threat to survival between 15 and 30 years of age

C are higher in coal-mining and quarrying than in any other occupational group outside the armed forces

D show no overlap in characteristics with those from suicide

E are higher at home than they are at work

4.10   Adverse drug reactions

A   are usually reported by the patient
B   are reliably and routinely notified by practising doctors
C   are a major cause of hospital morbidity
D   also occur to 'natural' and 'ethnic' medicaments
E   can be monitored effectively through cause-specific mortality rates

4.11   Leukaemia

A   incidence shows a definite occupational and social class pattern
B   mortality rates have increased over the last 40 years
C   prognosis has been unaffected by advances in treatment
D   incidence rates correlate well with geographical variation in background radiation
E   risk is increased after exposure to heavy radiation

4.12   Bladder cancer incidence is increased in

A   sufferers from bilharzia (Schistosoma haematobium)
B   cigarette smokers
C   dye factory workers exposed to beta naphthylamine
D   ladies' hairdressers
E   patients treated with cyclophosphamide

4.13   The NHS was formed in 1948 and

A   there was no Medical Officer of Health before this
B   all medical care before 1948 was private
C   brought all health services under one authority
D   was reorganized in 1974
E   general practitioner services were administered with the hospital services

4.14   Primary health care

A   is provided in the UK by general practitioners
B   is more adequately provided in most developing countries than hospital services
C   can only be provided by adequately trained doctors
D   is more expensive than hospital health care
E   is funded by local government in the UK

4.15   For it to be worth providing a screening service for a disease it is important

A   to use the best available test
B   to have a test with a low proportion of false negatives
C   that the disease has a high prevalence
D   that the disease has a high incidence
E   that the detected disease cases are readily treatable

4.16 Decisions on priorities in health care
  A   are necessary because resources are limited
  B   on how a service should be provided can be examined by
      cost effectiveness analysis
  C   on which service to provide can be examined by cost benefit
      analysis
  D   are difficult because it is difficult to measure health care input
  E   with immediate benefits are preferable to those which have
      delayed benefits

4.17 Social class
  A   gradient in mortality rate is a common finding
  B   grouping is determined by level of income
  C   inequality in health care is the subject of the Black report
  D   of married women is usually based on that of the husband
  E   categorization of doctors and ministers of the church is class I

4.18 Acute rheumatic fever
  A   and chronic rheumatic heart disease are the commonest
      forms of heart disease in developing countries
  B   is rare in developed countries
  C   can follow scarlet fever
  D   results in rheumatic heart disease only if it is recurrent
  E   can be positively diagnosed without laboratory evidence of
      staphylococcal infection

4.19 Rabies
  A   has been kept out of Britain largely because it is an island
  B   is a pathogen only of man, dogs and foxes
  C   vaccine is given routinely to certain Customs and Excise staff
  D   infection has a case fatality rate of around 50%
  E   vaccine is routinely given to travellers to the Indian
      subcontinent

4.20 Food poisoning
  A   with Bacillus cereus is usually associated with rice
  B   with Campylobacter is usually associated with milk
  C   with Campylobacter is characterized by abdominal pain
  D   is preventable by good standards of food hygiene
  E   from a catering establishment can result in prosecution under
      existing powers in the UK

4.21 Sewage

  A disposal is more expensive in coastal than inland cities
  B disposal in septic tanks has no place in developed countries
  C from humans is used in the form of slurry as a fertilizer on agricultural land
  D disposal systems can be used to track down carriers of Salmonella typhi
  E treatment is usually by chemical processing

4.22 An example of primary prevention is

  A measles immunization
  B cervical cytology screening
  C self examination of the breast for lumps
  D smoking cessation after a heart attack
  E fluoridation of water supply to prevent dental caries

Paper Four — Answers

4.1 **A True**   This is the commonest definition but sometimes the ratio used is with that in the population as a whole. For continuously distributed variables, such as blood pressure or serum cholesterol, the relative risk is the ratio between that in a particular risk-factor grouping and that in the lowest grouping, but the ratio of any two rates may be used.

    B True   Relative risk is widely used in studies of disease aetiology which are concerned with demonstrating associations and whether they are likely to be causal. The higher the relative risk the more likely the association is to be causal, provided it is very unlikely to have occurred by chance.

    C False   Case-control studies are widely used to estimate relative risk.

    D True   Attributable risk is the risk difference rather than the risk ratio. Attributable risk therefore says how much a risk difference matters in absolute rather than relative terms.

    E True   The relative risk for death from coronary disease in a heavy smoker is twice that in a non-smoker and the attributable risk is very high; for lung cancer the relative risk is 30 times but the attributable risk is rather lower. The reason for this is that the risk of lung cancer in the non-smoker is very low while that for coronary disease death is appreciable.

4.2 A **False**   Dead motor cyclists are a highly selected subset of all motorcyclists and this would assume that risk of death was evenly distributed.

    B **False**   This may be true but the evidence is insufficient without knowing the relative risk of death at different ages which would be based on death rates. These are calculated using the numbers of those at risk.

    C **False**   Again this may be true but the evidence is insufficient. It would be difficult to dissociate youth from the learning stage, in which an inexperienced driver may be accident prone.

    D **False**   No evidence for this.

    E **False**   Again there is no evidence for this without knowledge of the numbers at risk so that relative rates can be calculated.

4.3 A **False**   Although this is how epidemiology began, modern epidemiology is as much concerned with non-infectious diseases, such as cardiovascular disease, cancer and occupational disease, as it is with infections.

    B **False**   Epidemiological techniques are used to test causal hypotheses but the hypotheses themselves frequently do not come from epidemiological observations but from clinical observation or animal experiments.

    C **True**   This definition is worth remembering as it introduces the idea of a population based science, concerned with measurement of disease rates and study of risk factors.

    D **True**   Epidemiological studies are easier to carry out on common conditions but certain techniques, such as the case-control study, can be and are carried out on rare diseases.

    E **False**   It is doubtful that anyone trying these multiple choice questions will make this mistake, but it is amazing how often mail for the epidemiology department is found with the spelling of 'epidermiology' on it or arrives with a note saying 'try skin department'.

4.4 A **False**   The simple answer to this question is that age and sex standardization of mortality rates overcomes differences in these factors and enables valid comparisons to be made. The honours viva candidate might then add that standardization does not always remove the effect of these factors completely.

     B **True**   Major revision of the International Classification of Diseases may cause major discontinuities in disease trends. Major changes last occurred in 1968 and a minor change occurred in 1979 or 1980 in most countries.

     C **True**   Some diseases are much more likely to be detected at necropsy and whether one is done or not will depend on the current medico-legal practice. For example, sudden death from aortic stenosis or hypertrophic cardiomyopathy is likely to be ascribed to coronary heart disease unless there is a necropsy.

     D **True**   For example, there is a current fashion for putting death from coronary heart disease down to ventricular fibrillation which was previously ascribed to acute myocardial infarction, and two generations ago to angina pectoris or coronary spasm or degenerative heart disease. Diseases often stay within the same broader category (ischaemic or coronary heart disease or stroke), when the more specific category changes.

     E **True**   In many countries a significant proportion of deaths are ascribed to vague diagnoses or symptoms such as senility. If the rules are changed there is a risk that these cases will gravitate to convenient and unchallengeable diagnoses like myocardial infarction or pneumonia, especially in the elderly.

4.5 A **False**   The proportion of cases that end fatally within a defined time period is likely to be independent of the incidence rate.

     B **True**   The proportion of the population that has the disease will be increased by improved survival or by slower recovery or cure rates.

     C **True**   In the extreme all new cases die, and the incidence rate and mortality rate are then identical.

     D **False**   The rate at which new cases appear in those previously unaffected will not be affected by what happens to cases subsequently.

     E **False**   In epidemiological parlance the mortality rate is the death rate from the disease in a defined population group while the fatality rate is that among cases of the disease. The only occasion in which they could be identical would be if the whole population had got a disease.

4.6 A **True**   Where cases and controls are individually matched it
                         is common practice for each case to be matched with
                         a fixed number of controls but this can be more than
                         one. Where there is a small number of cases there are
                         definite advantages in having a larger number of
                         controls. There is also an advantage in having more
                         than one group of controls chosen in different ways.

    B **False**   Cases and controls should be matched for factors
                         whose effect is to be eliminated as of no interest (such
                         as age and sex). Matching should not be done for
                         factors that are to be investigated.

    C **True**   Relative risk can be calculated from the relative
                         frequency with which the risk-factor is present in
                         cases versus controls or by pair matching, from the
                         frequency with which matched pairs are discordant
                         for the presence of the factor.

    D **True**   As the disease has already developed in the cases,
                         information on the presence of the suspected risk-
                         factors is retrospective and therefore subject to
                         potential bias.

    E **False**   The case-control study is the only epidemiological
                         design that allows the investigation of rare diseases,
                         as these will not occur often enough to figure as
                         prevalence cases in a cross-sectional study, or as
                         incidence cases in a cohort (longitudinal) study.

4.7 A **False** The most effective way of lowering serum cholesterol is to lower the proportion of food energy obtained from certain saturated fats, perhaps substituting some polyunsaturated fats which have a mild cholesterol lowering effect. The effect of dietary cholesterol is weaker and more controversial, and a reduction in dietary cholesterol without a change in saturated fats will have a much smaller effect.

B **False** Some vegetable fats are saturated and margarine may be made industrially by catalytic hydrogenation of polyunsaturated vegetable fats to make saturated fats. Fats from ruminant animals (sheep and cattle) are very saturated, while those from pigs, poultry and game are less saturated; fish oils contain a relatively high polyunsaturated component.

C **False** The recommended reduction in food energy from saturated fats should be replaced by other foods of which the complex carbohydrates of vegetables and fruit are thought to be advantageous.

D **True** The serum cholesterol of most people will fall as a result of the application of a cholesterol lowering diet. Failure is more likely to be caused by failure to comply than from any metabolic resistance.

E **True** There has been no large-scale randomized controlled trial of diet alone in the prevention of coronary heart disease. Pilot studies done in the US in the 1960s suggested that any such study would be extremely expensive and difficult to carry out.

4.8 A **True** Unlike coronary heart disease, which shows a strong male excess, stroke death rates in the two sexes are similar. In some countries there is a male excess and in other countries a female one.

B **True** Blood pressure is the most consistent and powerful risk factor for stroke. Serum cholesterol and smoking appear to be risk factors in some studies but not in others.

C **True** Stroke is common in countries like Japan and China, in the Caribbean countries and in Africa, where coronary heart disease is rare.

D **False** More stroke survivors die from heart disease than from stroke.

E **False** Although some stroke victims remain hemiplegic, perhaps a half recover completely, so that a prevalence survey would not detect them.

4.9 A **True**   Males are more accident prone from the time they are toddlers right through to old age. More elderly women have accidents but there are far more elderly women around.

B **True**   Accidents account for a small proportion of the total of all deaths, but in the age groups in which death rates are at their lowest, accidents are the predominant cause of death.

C **False**   Deep sea fishing is more dangerous, but the statistics used to be incomplete through failure to register deaths outside territorial waters.

D **False**   A large number of deaths which are classified as accidental are probably suicide, but there is insufficient evidence to be certain. The circumstances, nature, and age and sex distribution of these doubtful cases closely resemble those for suicide.

E **True**   Although many occupations are hazardous most people spend far more time at home than at work and accident rates are higher overall.

4.10 A **False**   Patients may consider them to be part of the disease or may be shy about reporting them (e.g. impotence).

B **False**   Doctors report a small percentage of adverse drug reactions; despite a 'yellow card' system of notification in Britain. Special systems have to be established for monitoring all adverse reactions in a particular context.

C **True**   About 10% of hospital admissions are complicated by drug reactions and one estimate is that 3% of hospital admissions are occasioned by them.

D **True**   Any drug is potentially dangerous and many Third World treatments contain heavy metals or other poisons. The only exception to the general rule might be homeopathic remedies that are prescribed at such low doses that the risk of adverse reactions must also be correspondingly small.

E **False**   Deaths are usually attributed to the disease being treated rather than the remedy, even if the latter was dangerous. Adverse reactions accounted for 92 000 hospital discharges in England and Wales in 1980 but the mortality statistics only attributed 10 deaths to this cause, whereas many more deaths must have been precipitated or hastened by adverse reactions to drugs.

4.11 A False There is no clear association and therefore no clues to aetiology from this source.

B True Leukaemia mortality rates are changing relatively faster than those for most other forms of malignancy but it is not a common cause of death ($< 1\%$).

C False Prognosis in certain sorts of leukaemia has been dramatically changed by the advent of intensive cytotoxic therapy.

D False Despite the known association of leukaemia with high radiation levels, no association has been found with the low levels of naturally occurring radiation, which vary considerably and are determined by the geology of the locality.

E True This association was recognized from the atomic bomb survivors and also from those given therapeutic spinal irradiation to control ankylosing spondylitis. The excess risk declines after a period of years.

4.12 A True The bladder is damaged by the parasite, and malignancy supervenes.

B True There is an increased risk, presumably from concentration of excreted carcinogens in the bladder.

C True Cohorts of chemical factory workers followed from their exposure many years ago show a very high proportion developing bladder cancer.

D True Again, dyes or other substances used by hairdressers may be involved.

E True Chemical cystitis may go on to malignancy.

4.13 A False The first Medical Officers of Health were appointed in the 19th century and the post was firmly established in public health services long before the formation of the NHS.

B False The formation of the NHS in 1948 was the culmination of a series of developments in health care provision. Public hospital care was provided by local authorities prior to 1948.

C False The organization of the NHS as set up in 1948 was tripartite in form. The three parts were the hospital service, administered by Hospital Boards, the general practitioner service administered by Executive Councils and the public health service, administered by local government.

D True Reorganization of the NHS in 1974 brought the three parts under one authority, i.e. hospitals, primary care and public health. Environmental health was left under local government control.

E False The primary care and hospitals were kept as separate services under the NHS in 1948.

4.14 A **True**   General practitioners, in conjunction with health visitors and district nurses, provide primary care services in the UK.

B **False**   The reverse is true; most developing countries have hospitals but many lack adequate primary health care.

C **False**   Primary health care can be provided by different personnel such as paramedical workers and basic health workers.

D **False**   Hospital services are far more costly than primary health care.

E **False**   Primary health care is funded by health authorities.

4.15 A **False**   The requirements for a good screening test are different from those for a good diagnostic test. A screening test should be cheap, reliable and acceptable to a large number of people.

B **True**   Although a screening service can be justified in terms of its cost in relation to those it benefits, which may only be some of the potential cases, there is an implied promise to the public that disease cases will be identified. False negatives from a screening are lost and cannot be picked up and they may be given a false sense of security, which may even delay their diagnosis. False positives, however, will be alarmed by the recall letter, but their true status will be discovered when a definitive diagnostic procedure is performed.

C **True**   Screening is only applicable for diseases with a high prevalence rates, the return when screening for rare conditions is very low.

D **False**   The prevalence of disease but not necessarily the incidence should be high. Where the incidence is high and duration short it is very difficult for screening to detect cases.

E **True**   There is no point in screening to detect early disease if nothing can be done about the cases detected. There must be an effective intervention and the resources must be available locally to provide it expeditiously to those picked up by the screening service.

4.16 A **True**   When there is no limit to resources the health service can do all that it wishes to do. Only when these resources are finite do choices have to be made.

    B **True**   Cost effectiveness analysis examines different ways of providing a service. The least cost for a given objective, or the greatest output for a fixed budget, can be examined in cost effectiveness analysis.

    C **True**   Where a variety of options are available for consideration, cost benefit analysis is employed to determine which service would give the greatest benefit for the resources available.

    D **False**   Input, i.e. expenditure of money and staff time, are relatively easy to measure. Choices in health care are difficult because it is difficult to measure the output of services.

    E **True**   Instant benefit for expenditure is preferred to delayed benefit because the future is uncertain and the value of benefits in the future is less because of discounting. Health education benefits are usually long-term.

4.17 A **True**   The mortality rates in the lower social classes are usually found to be higher than those for the higher social classes.

    B **False**   Social class is determined by occupation. The occupations are classed by their apparent standing in the community, not by their level of income.

    C **True**   The Black report on inequalities in health care is largely concerned with the lack of health care provision to the lower social classes.

    D **True**   It has been found that the social class grouping of husbands is much more stable than that for their wives so the social class of married women is usually based on their husband's occupation.

    E **True**   Doctors, solicitors and ministers are in social class I. Teachers and nurses are in II. Unskilled workers are V.

4.18 A **True**   Rheumatic heart disease is by far the most common heart disease in developing countries.

B **True**   Acute rheumatic fever is now very rare in developed countries although the reason for this is not clear. Most of the decline occurred before the advent of antibiotics.

C **True**   Scarlet fever and acute rheumatic fever are both associated with streptococcal infection.

D **False**   The likelihood of rheumatic heart disease is more common if there are recurrent episodes of acute rheumatic fever but it may follow a single episode; many patients with rheumatic heart disease have no history of acute rheumatic fever.

E **True**   Acute rheumatic fever usually follows streptococcal, not staphylococcal infection, and the Jones diagnostic criteria include preceding evidence of a streptococcal infection.

4.19 A **True**   The most important factor in keeping rabies out of Britain is that it is surrounded by water. Strict control of importation of animals is thus more easy to maintain. Once rabies is endemic in an animal population it is very hard to eradicate.

B **False**   Rabies also affects many biting mammals including cats, mongooses and bats. Bats are a reservoir of rabies in America and Europe.

C **True**   The rabies vaccine is routinely given to protect Customs and Excise staff who deal with animal importation. A three dose primary course is given and a single booster dose every two years.

D **False**   The case fatality from rabies infection is virtually 100%.

E **False**   Post exposure vaccination is recommended for travellers; pre-exposure vaccination is only given to a few individuals in high risk employment.

4.20 A **True**   Bacillus cereus food poisoning is usually associated with rice and in particular fried rice.

B **True**   Campylobacter infection is often associated with unpasteurized milk supplies but can also be water borne or from poultry.

C **True**   Abdominal pain, diarrhoea, vomiting and fever are the characteristic symptoms of Campylobacter infection.

D **True**   Most episodes of food poisoning are due to poor food handling and are preventable by good standards of food hygiene.

E **True**   Wide powers exist under present legislation in the UK and other countries to prosecute and close down immediately premises which present a risk to the public.

4.21 A **False**   Cities on the coast can discharge sewage into the sea whereas inland areas require to treat their sewage before discharging into water courses.

     B **False**   In rural areas septic tanks are widely used as an efficient and inexpensive method of sewage disposal.

     C **True**   Although human sewage can be used as a fertilizer there are certain restrictions on spraying slurry near harvesting.

     D **True**   Sewerage systems have often been used to track down carriers of Salmonella typhi by using sewer swabs at different points through the system.

     E **False**   Chemical processing of sewage is rarely used; sewage is usually biologically degraded.

4.22 A **True**   Normal, healthy children are immunized to prevent measles infection.

     B **False**   Cervical smears are examined for early evidence of disease. Prevention of progression to overt disease is known as secondary prevention.

     C **False**   Self examination only finds existing disease early and does not prevent breast cancer.

     D **False**   Prevention of recurrences is secondary not primary prevention. Prevention of recurrence or complications of overt disease is called tertiary prevention.

     E **True**   Fluoride is incorporated into teeth and primarily prevents occurrence of caries.

Paper Five — Questions

5.1 In a case-control study

A there need not be equal numbers of men and women
B cases and controls should be matched for all possible factors
C controls should be free of any known disease
D there must be equal numbers of cases and controls
E history of exposure to risk factors should be elicited without knowledge of whether the subject is a case or a control

5.2 In a country where there was no legislation on the subject a survey of car drivers killed in road accidents showed that half of them were wearing seat belts. It can be concluded that

A not all car drivers wear seat belts
B seat belts reduce the risk of a fatal accident by half
C only half of car drivers wear seat belts
D seat belts do not give complete protection from fatal injury
E a control series of drivers who survive major accidents is needed

5.3 Mortality in different populations may be compared validly by

A age- and sex-specific mortality rates
B indirectly age-standardized mortality rates
C mean age at death
D directly age-standardized mortality rates
E levels of life insurance claims

5.4 Over the last 20 years there has been an increase in the Standardized Mortality Ratio (SMR) for a certain cancer. Possible explanations include

A the increase in the age of the population
B the decrease in deaths from infectious disease means that more people die of cancer
C the cancer was previously misdiagnosed more frequently than now
D there has been an improvement in survival times
E the incidence rate has increased

5.5   A satirical review once based a comedy sketch on the observation that being a judge is safer than being a coalminer, because there is less danger from falling coal. In order to compare overall occupational risk you could use

A   numbers of coalminers and judges seen in a hospital accident and emergency department

B   standardized mortality ratios (SMRs)

C   age-specific death rates

D   percentage of coalminers and judges who die while at work

E   reported age at death in newspaper reports

5.6   Epidemiological measures of mortality in a population are interrelated so that

A   the crude mortality rate is the mean of the age-specific rates for all ages

B   the infant mortality rate is the sum of the perinatal mortality rate and the post-neonatal mortality rate

C   if the SMRs for both men and women in a locality are 100 it means that they have the same life expectancy

D   an SMR of 120 means that the death rate is 120 per 100 000 per year

E   a male life expectancy of 72 means that men aged 65 have an average of only seven years to live and men aged 70 only two years

5.7   The relationship between blood pressure and coronary risk

A   is true both for systolic and diastolic blood pressure

B   has been shown to be reversible by treatment of hypertension

C   extends throughout the range of blood pressure readings

D   is such that most coronary events from raised blood pressure occur when it is very high

E   disappears in men reaching the age of 60

5.8   In the medical care of cardiovascular disease

A   stroke accounts for fewer hospital admissions than myocardial infarction

B   stroke victims occupy more hospital beds than do victims of myocardial infarction

C   once hypertension is detected, 90% of it is effectively treated

D   hypertension cases are best first investigated and treated in hospital rather than by general practitioners

E   risk of death for the first year after myocardial infarction can be reduced by drug therapy

5.9   Suicide

A   is commoner in women than men
B   occurs most commonly in young adults
C   declined in Britain during the 1960s and 1970s
D   risk is unrelated to ease of access to means of self-destruction
E   can occur in epidemics

5.10   Carcinoma of the stomach

A   is declining as a cause of death in most Western countries
B   survival beyond five years is exceptional
C   is commoner in professional than manual workers
D   death rates are greatest in the 55–64 age group
E   is commoner in those with blood group A

5.11   With respect to occupational lung disease

A   bird fanciers' lung is the lay term for ornithosis contracted from pigeons
B   asbestos causes mesothelioma less commonly than pulmonary fibrosis
C   chronic brochitis is a notifiable occupational disease of postal delivery workers
D   silicosis hazards are reduced by water spraying
E   chest radiograph findings correlate well with levels of disability

5.12   Licensing regulations concerned with road safety allow you to drive a

A   heavy goods vehicle if your epilepsy has been controlled by drugs for one year
B   public service vehicle if your myopia is corrected by glasses
C   farm tractor for ploughing if you have paranoid schizophrenia
D   heavy goods vehicle if you have maturity onset diabetes controlled by diet
E   car if you have had a myocardial infarct three months ago

5.13   Management in health authorities

A   is by elected officials
B   is responsible to the Secretary of State
C   is under the authority of a medical officer
D   has responsibility for school health services
E   has responsibility for Social Work Departments

5.14 New developments in the health services
A   can be assessed by marginal analysis
B   can be assessed by cost benefit analysis
C   are routinely assessed by multiple regression analysis
D   often save money
E   are often creeping and unplanned

5.15 A suitable screening test for
A   diabetes is the glucose tolerance test
B   disease should be cheap and acceptable
C   early disease should have a high coverage in those at risk
D   early breast cancer is self examination of breasts
E   phenylketonuria is routinely performed in the UK

5.16 The size of a population
A   largely determines its need of health care
B   is largely determined by the birth rate
C   is calculated by the General Household Survey
D   is calculated in some countries from a population register
E   can be calculated from the electoral register

5.17 The 1974 reorganization of the NHS
A   coincided with a reorganization in local government
B   divided the service into three parts
C   brought the Medical Officer of Health into the local
     government service
D   changed Environmental Health Departments from the health
     service to local government
E   brought the general practitioner services under the health
     authorities

5.18 Plague
A   is endemic in rodents in the USA
B   is endemic in rodents in India
C   was controlled in London by the work of John Snow
D   has an incubation period of two to eight weeks
E   can be transmitted in droplets

5.19 Hepatitis
A   prophylaxis with human immunoglobulin should be given at
     least four weeks before travel to India
B   prophylaxis with human immunoglobulin is effective against
     both hepatitis A and hepatitis B
C   B has a case fatality of 50%
D   A is transmitted by the faecal-oral route
E   A is more common in children and young adults than in older
     age groups

5.20 In good food handling practice
- **A** larger frozen fowls should be allowed to defrost longer than small ones
- **B** defrosting poultry should be kept at the bottom of the refrigerator
- **C** all staff should be screened for carriage of Salmonella
- **D** staff excreting Campylobacter should be excluded from work until they are stool culture negative
- **E** milk should be boiled for 10 minutes

5.21 A safe water supply
- **A** alone would have little effect on disease in developing countries
- **B** from recycled supplies should be free from bacteria and viruses
- **C** is simply a matter of keeping water supply separate from sewage
- **D** usually contains chlorine to inhibit bacterial growth
- **E** is acidified to limit the solubility of lead

5.22 The routine prevention programme in the UK includes
- **A** rubella immunization for all school children
- **B** typhoid immunization for food handlers
- **C** regular chest x-ray for pathology technicians
- **D** diphtheria immunization in the first year of life
- **E** smallpox vaccination for all virology department staff

Paper Five — Answers

5.1   A **True**   Sexual equality has not been carried this far and the disease under investigation may be specific to one sex!

      B **False**   If you match for a factor you cannot investigate its contribution as a risk-factor. You must therefore match for factors you wish to eliminate from consideration which could confound the result, e.g. age and sex. Other factors depend on the context (social class, area of residence, race, parity, etc.) The more factors you want to match for, the bigger the choice of controls needs to be.

      C **False**   Controls should be free of the disease under investigation but in many studies patients have been used who were suffering from other conditions. This can introduce biases and it is necessary to use patients with diseases of different kinds so that their risk factors do not influence the result too much.

      D **False**   There are often equal numbers, especially when cases and controls have been pair matched. However, if the number of cases is small it is advisable to have more controls and in many studies there are several control groups chosen in different ways.

      E **True**   The major problems with this sort of study are in the choice of controls and the possibility of bias in ascertainment of risk-factor exposure between cases and controls.

5.2 A **True**   If all drivers wore belts, all drivers killed would be wearing belts.

B **False**   There is insufficient evidence without knowledge of the prevalence of belt wearing either in survivors or motorists generally.

C **False**   This would only be true if wearing had no effect on survival.

D **True**   Or no-one who died would be wearing one.

E **True**   A control series of survivors would indicate the degree of benefit of wearing a belt for those involved in a major accident. However, critics of seat belts at one time argued that they caused accidents, and to confirm or deny this a study would be needed of the prevalence of belt wearing among all drivers, the prevalence among those involved in any accident and the prevalence among those killed in accidents. This would show whether belt wearing influences the risk of having an accident and also the risk of surviving an accident.

5.3 A **True**   This is what these rates are for.

B **True**   Indirect age standardization results in the commonly used indicator of comparative mortality known as the SMR or standardized mortality ratio which gives a value of 100 to the standard population. Rates for the standard population are applied to the index population to obtain an expected number of deaths and the observed number is expressed as a percentage of this.

C **False**   Mean age at death is likely to be affected too much by the age structure of the population, which results from past patterns of fertility and migration, which will distort the effect of mortality rates alone.

D **True**   Here the age-specific rates from the index population are applied to the standard (e.g. European or world) population to see what the overall rate for a broad age group would have been had the age structure been the same as that for the standard.

E **False**   Early epidemiology was based on life insurance results, but there are three major biases. The majority of the population never take out life insurance, some individuals take out several policies so that they appear more than once, and a large proportion of policies are allowed to lapse so that the fate of the insured is never known. Claims experience is therefore biased by these factors.

5.4 A **False** The purpose of age standardization is to take out the effect of changes in the age structure of the population.

B **False** This is a common fallacy. Everyone has to die of something so that fewer deaths from one cause means more from other causes. However, if age-specific death rates from certain causes diminish there is no necessary increase in age-specific rates (or age-standardized rates) for other causes. The population will live slightly longer. A larger number of people will live to an older age so that for the same death rate per thousand in that older age group a larger number will die.

C **True** Some of the increase in mortality rates from internal cancers in this century may be because of better diagnosis. It is useful if it can be shown what the previous mistaken diagnosis was as this should be diminished.

D **False** An improvement in survival time means that survivors have a greater chance of living long enough to contract other serious diseases so that the original cancer will be less likely to appear on their death certificates. Therefore mortality rates will fall.

E **True** Of course this is the simplest explanation and one that is most commonly assumed when trends are being looked at, but other explanations should also be considered.

5.5 A **False** It is unlikely that the same hospital would serve both coalmines and the lawcourts except in certain towns; numbers of hospital attendances would have to be converted to rates to take account of the different numbers of coalminers and judges.

B **True** This would be a basis for comparison although there would be difficulties in that many coalminers would have stopped working at the coalface by the age that most judges are appointed.

C **True** The comparison would be valid if there were sufficient overlap of ages.

D **False** This comparison would be confounded by the effect of age. Most miners would die at work from accidents while judges would die from diseases associated with increasing age.

E **False** The death of an elderly judge is likely to be reported, while that of coalminers would not be reported routinely. Age at death is a poor indicator of comparative risk because of the very different age distribution of the two groups. Judges tend to die as judges; coalminers retire into other jobs and their occupational history may not be reported.

5.6 A **False** The crude mortality rate reflects the different contributions made by different numbers at risk at different ages in a given population, whereas age-specific rates will have the same sized denominator.

B **False** The perinatal mortality rate includes still births, while infant mortality rate does not, and it stops at one week after birth rather than 28 days which is when the post-neotal period starts. The infant mortality rate (deaths from live births in the first year) does equal the sum of the neonatal and the post-neonatal mortality rate.

C **False** If the SMRs for both men and women are 100 it means that they are both at their expected level. Female death rates in general are considerably lower than those for men at all ages, so that the expected rate for women, derived from a female standard population, will be lower than that for men, derived from a male population.

D **False** It means that there are 120 deaths occurring for every 100 predicted from the rates in the standard population, and these could have almost any value as a rate per 100 000 per year.

E **False** The number of years you can expect to live diminishes less than one year for every year that you live, so that you always have a positive expectation of life, even when you have lived beyond the average. This is because those who have already died no longer figure in the calculations.

5.7 **A True** Both systolic and diastolic blood pressure are risk-factors for coronary heart disease and there is a very high correlation between them. If anything, systolic blood pressure is the better predictor but this is argued.

B False Unfortunately there is no good evidence from randomized controlled trials that treatment of mild and moderate hypertension lowers coronary risk, although strokes and other cardiovascular end-points are substantially diminished.

C True There is no good evidence of a threshold below which levels of blood pressure are of no importance. It seems more likely that there is a gradient throughout the whole range, although this is curvilinear so that the slope increases at higher levels.

D False Although the risk to the individual is at a maximum at the highest levels of blood pressure, the number of individuals affected is very small, whereas the number of individuals with average or slightly above average pressures is enormous. This latter group accounts for the majority of blood pressure related coronary events.

E False Blood pressure continues to be a major coronary risk factor through the 60s age group.

5.8 **A True** Myocardial infarction is a commoner cause of hospital admission than stroke. Stroke tends to occur in the elderly and myocardial infarction cases are commoner in middle age.

B True Length of stay for a myocardial infarction is 6–12 days depending on the hospital, but severe stroke cases may need nursing for many weeks or even months, occupying both acute medical and long-stay beds, so that strokes are a heavy drain on nursing resources.

C False Studies in the early 1970s in the USA suggested that only half of the hypertension that had been detected was treated and only half of that was adequately treated. Major campaigns in the USA have improved these figures in some centres. British studies suggest that high blood pressure readings are often ignored and that unless the problem is treated systematically many victims will not be adequately treated.

D False The great majority of mild and moderate hypertension of middle-age can be managed in general practice. Hospital hypertension clinics can be sent the young, unusual, severe or refractory cases, and undertake research.

E True Beta blocker therapy has been shown in large trials to reduce the risk of fatal recurrence when started after myocardial infarction.

5.9 A **False**   Suicide is twice as common in men, although overdoses and other similar gestures short of completed suicide are commoner in women.

B **False**   Rates are highest in older people, where they are associated with mental illness, alcoholism, bereavement, loneliness and despair. Those associated with serious disease are often attributed to the disease, so that they are concealed.

C **True**   Suicide rates overall declined while that from most specific methods of committing suicide increased. The decline in coal-gas poisoning was so great that it outweighed the increase in the others.

D **False**   The coal-gas story above, the very high suicide rate in the USA from gunshot wounds, and the high rate of suicidal drug overdosage in Britain among doctors, nurses and (most importantly because the first two like to say how stressful their work is) pharmacists, all suggest that the ready availability of the means and the knowledge of how to use them are major contributors to suicide risk.

E **True**   There are many recorded examples. An outbreak of young lovers throwing themselves into a Japanese volcano had to be stopped by force; Marilyn Monroe's suicide was widely copied all over America; mass suicides of religious sects have been reported and reports of individuals publicly pouring petrol over themselves and setting light to it led to so many imitations that the British media agreed to stop further reports.

5.10 A **True**   As treatment is relatively ineffective, there must have been a real decline in incidence in many countries, presumably from a change in environmental factors or lifestyle.

B **True**   Incidence rates and mortality rates are almost identical.

C **False**   There is, as for so many diseases, a positive social class gradient with an excess of deaths in unskilled and semi-skilled workers and their wives.

D **False**   As for most cancers, rates rise exponentially with age.

E **True**   There is a 20% excess; enough to be interesting but not to cause alarm and despondency in the 40% of the population with group A!

5.11 A **False**   Bird fanciers' lung belongs to the same family as farmers' lung, called allergic extrinsic alveolitis, whereas ornithosis is a viral pneumonia caught from birds.

B **True**   Although mesothelioma is very specific for asbestos and other mineral fibres, it is comparatively rare, while respiratory impairment from exposure to asbestos dust is more common.

C **False**   Although the association with outdoor working was demonstrated in postal workers in the 1950s, the major risk factor for chronic bronchitis is cigarette smoking and it is not recognized as an industrial disease.

D **True**   Wherever it is possible to control silica dust at source, by spraying it with water, the risk will be correspondingly reduced.

E **False**   While radiographic evidence helps with the confirmation of the diagnosis for lung diseases, in some, such as pulmonary fibrosis, the degree of disability may be quite disproportionate to the radiographic appearance.

5.12 A **False**   Epilepsy has to be completely controlled by drugs for three years before an ordinary driving licence can be considered, and it is an absolute contra-indication to holding a heavy goods or public service.

B **True**   If corrected eyesight is adequate, the fact of wearing glasses is not important although a spare pair should be carried on long journeys. Very severe myopoia (six dioptres) may be considered a contra-indication to taking up driving as a career.

C **True**   There are no restrictions on what is driven by whom off the public roads, whether or not it is a good idea.

D **True**   Diabetes controlled by diet is unlikely to lead to hypoglycaemic attack or other sudden incapacity although the driver should be warned of symptoms of diabetic pre-coma.

E **True**   There are no restrictions on holding an ordinary driving licence with coronary heart disease provided that it is not within three months of a myocardial infarction, nor with angina pectoris provoked by driving. It is not permitted to drive a heavy goods vehicle or public service vehicle with diagnosed coronary heart disease.

5.13 A **False**   The management of health authorities is by boards, members of which are nominated by the Secretary of State. The boards appoint officers to carry out work for them.

B **True**   Ultimately, health authorities are the responsibility of the Secretary of State and his Department of Health.

C **False**   Health authorities are managed by boards and their officers. While these officers include medical officers they are not in overall authority.

D **True**   Health authorities provide school health services to bring about regular examinations of pupils and immunization.

E **False**   Social Work Departments are responsible to local government, not to the health authority.

5.14 A **True**   Marginal analysis is an appropriate method of assessing new developments. It looks at the change in cost and the change in benefits.

B **True**   In cost benefit analysis the benefit of a new service is estimated and compared with the cost of providing it.

C **False**   Multiple regression is a statistical technique used in research and it is not routinely used for this purpose.

D **False**   Few new developments save money, most increase expenditure on health services.

E **True**   Many new developments occur without any planning or decision to fund them.

5.15 A **False**   Glucose tolerance tests are a useful diagnostic procedure but are not appropriate for screening as they are time consuming. A single fasting blood glucose estimation or a test for glycosuria would be more appropriate.

B **True**   Along with reliability and validity, screening tests should be cheap and acceptable.

C **True**   It is essential that those at risk are screened. However, it often is the case that those at greatest risk are hardest to screen.

D **True**   Self examination is a method of screening for early breast lumps. Examination by a trained observer is better but is obviously more expensive.

E **True**   Blood or urine is tested in the neonatal period for phenylketonuria in the UK.

5.16 A **False**   The size of a population only in part determines its need of health care; the age structure and morbidity experience are the major determinants of need.

    B **False**   The size of population is determined by births, deaths and migration, and not only by the birth rate. Population growth is more closely related to the birth rate.

    C **False**   The General Household Survey is a sample survey based on households. It does not measure population size.

    D **True**   The Netherlands and Scandinavian countries maintain population registers from which information on population size and character can be obtained.

    E **False**   Not everybody in a community is listed in the electoral register. Those under voting age are not included, nor are those who have recently moved into an area.

5.17 A **True**   The boundaries for health districts, areas and regions were aligned with local government in 1974.

    B **False**   The 1974 reorganization brought an existing tripartite health service of hospitals, primary care and public health under one authority.

    C **False**   Before 1974 the Medical Officer of Health was part of the local government organization. In 1974 the Medical Officer of Health post was done away with and the duties were divided up between local government services and the health authority.

    D **False**   The Environmental Health Departments were formed in 1974. Prior to this their work was performed by the Department of the Medical Officer of Health.

    E **True**   Prior to 1974 the general practitioners came under a separate authority. In 1974 general practitioners, hospitals and community health services all came under the health authority.

5.18 A **True**   Wild rodent plague is known to exist in the western third of the USA so that plague is a potential danger to humans in that area.

    B **True**   Wild rodent plague is also known to exist in India and most of Asia, and in Central and South America.

    C **False**   John Snow's work was mainly concerned with cholera transmission from water supplies.

    D **False**   Plague has a short incubation period of two to six days.

    E **True**   While bites from infected fleas are the most common source of infection, airborne droplets are the next most common source. These droplets come from cases of plague pneumonia.

5.19 A False The effect of human immunoglobulin begins to wane immediately and so should be administered just prior to departure.

B False For prophylaxis against hepatitis B infection, hepatitis B immuno-globulin is required.

C False It is often thought that the case fatality from hepatitis B is very high but in fact it is quite low, probably less than 1%.

D True The faecal-oral route is the main means of transmission of hepatitis A.

E True Hepatitis A infection is rare in the older age groups.

5.20 A True Larger fowls take longer to defrost and if inadequately defrosted will be frozen at the centre on cooking, and pathogens will not be killed.

B True If defrosting poultry is put at the top of a refrigerator it will drip onto the food below, and contaminate foods which may not be cooked before consumption.

C False This practice is unnecessary; good food handling techniques are more important.

D False It is only necessary to exclude staff with Campylobacter infection while they are symptomatic. No routine follow-up stool tests are necessary.

E False In the pasteurization process milk can be heated to 63–66 °C for 30 minutes or 71 °C for 15 seconds. The milk then requires to be rapidly cooled to less than 10 °C to prevent multiplication of surviving organisms. Boiling of milk is not necessary and is likely to denature milk protein. The ultra heat treatment (UHT) method heats milk to 132 °C for one second.

5.21 A False A safe water supply would prevent the large number of water-borne diseases, which result in considerable morbidity and mortality in developing countries.

B False Safe water supplies are rarely free from bacteria. Recycled water supplies usually contain viruses which are not filtered or degraded in sewage treatment.

C True Water is made unsafe by contamination with sewage; keeping the two separate is the main problem.

D True Chlorine is added to water to prevent bacterial growth, as it acts as a disinfectant.

E False Lead is more soluble in acidic water so the pH of water requires to be raised to reduce the solubility of lead.

5.22 A **False**   Rubella immunization is only offered to girls in the UK. In the USA both boys and girls are given rubella vaccine in an attempt to eradicate the infection.

B **False**   Good food handling practice is much more important than immunization.

C **True**   This is carried out because pathology department staff are at risk of tuberculosis.

D **True**   Diphtheria vaccine is part of the standard triple vaccine given to children in the first year of life.

E **False**   Smallpox vaccine is now only given to staff of departments which hold the smallpox virus, and there are very few of these in the world.